Advance Praise for *The F*

"In *The Fibro Fix*, Dr. David Brady provides a comprehensive, strategic, easy-to-utilize plan to eliminate fibromyalgia's debilitating symptoms. Apply these principles and reclaim your life!"

—*JJ Virgin, CNS, CHFS, celebrity nutrition and fitness expert and bestselling author of* The Virgin Diet *and* JJ Virgin's Sugar Impact Diet

"*The Fibro Fix* is game changer and must-read for the millions of chronically ill patients who suffer from fibromyalgia and are failing under the conventional medical approach. Dr. Brady's program integrates the best of basic and clinical science through a cutting-edge functional medicine approach. Dr. David Brady is an internationally renowned expert in fibromyalgia, master nutritionist, scholar of natural medicine, VP of health sciences at the University of Bridgeport and compassionate healer. He has provided fibromyalgia patients a home run."

—*Gerard E. Mullin, MD, associate professor of medicine at The Johns Hopkins University School of Medicine and author of* The Gut Balance Revolution

"Dr. Brady takes his extensive knowledge and experience with fibromyalgia and gives readers a smart, holistic plan that treats the root cause of chronic pain and constant fatigue. Finally, a road map that will help so many people feel better immediately. This book is a game changer."

—*Susan S. Blum, MD, MPH, author of* The Immune System Recovery Plan *and founder and director of the Blum Center for Health*

"If you have fibromyalgia, chances are you have been misdiagnosed and misinformed at some point in your journey and are still suffering needlessly. With *The Fibro Fix*, help is here at last! Dr. David Brady unravels the puzzle of fibromyalgia with a comprehensive, individualized, and root-cause approach that can help you eliminate your pain and recover your health!"

—*Izabella Wentz, PharmD, author of the* New York Times *bestseller* Hashimoto's Thyroiditis

"This book is a must-read for anyone suffering from chronic pain. After years of helping people recover from fibromyalgia, Dr. David Brady has taken his clinical experience and made it accessible to those who may not be able to travel and see him. Dr. Brady's book can be thought of as a carefully crafted road map back to health. He helps you understand if you have fibromyalgia, what are the causes that give rise to it, and how you can reclaim your health in as little as 21 days. He helps you heal by sharing the most important steps for your diet, exercise, and supplementation. His approach is unique in that it focuses primarily on safe and nontoxic treatments. If you have chronic pain, carefully follow the steps in the book and share the references and use the well-referenced technical information to educate your physician."

—*Alan Christianson, NMD*, New York Times *bestselling author of*
The Adrenal Reset Diet

The

FIBRO
FIX

THE

FIBRO
FIX

GET TO THE ROOT OF YOUR
FIBROMYALGIA
AND START REVERSING
YOUR CHRONIC PAIN
AND FATIGUE IN 21 DAYS

DR. DAVID BRADY

RODALE.

This book is intended as a reference volume only, not as a medical manual. The information
given here is designed to help you make informed decisions about your health. It is not intended
as a substitute for any treatment that may have been prescribed by your doctor. If you suspect
that you have a medical problem, we urge you to seek competent medical help.

The information in this book is meant to supplement, not replace, proper exercise training.
All forms of exercise pose some inherent risks. The editors and publisher advise readers to take
full responsibility for their safety and know their limits. Before practicing the exercises in this
book, be sure that your equipment is well-maintained, and do not take risks beyond your level of
experience, aptitude, training, and fitness. The exercise and dietary programs in this book are not
intended as a substitute for any exercise routine or dietary regimen that may have been
prescribed by your doctor. As with all exercise and dietary programs, you should get your
doctor's approval before beginning.

Mention of specific companies, organizations, or authorities in this book does not imply
endorsement by the author or publisher, nor does mention of specific companies, organizations,
or authorities imply that they endorse this book, its author, or the publisher.

Internet addresses and telephone numbers given in this book were accurate
at the time it went to press.

© 2016 by David M. Brady, ND

Fibro-Fix™ is a trademark of Formulated Nutriceuticals, LLC.

All rights reserved. No part of this publication may be reproduced or transmitted in any form or
by any means, electronic or mechanical, including photocopying, recording, or any other
information storage and retrieval system, without the written permission of the publisher.

Rodale books may be purchased for business or promotional use
or for special sales. For information, please write to:
Special Markets Department, Rodale Inc., 733 Third Avenue, New York, NY 10017

Printed in the United States of America

Rodale Inc. makes every effort to use acid-free ♾, recycled paper ♻.

Illustrations by Paul Girard

Book design by Amy C. King

Library of Congress Cataloging-in-Publication Data is on file with the publisher.

ISBN 978-1-62336-712-1 paperback

Distributed to the trade by Macmillan

4 6 8 10 9 7 5 3   paperback

Follow us @RodaleBooks on

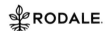
RODALE.

We inspire health, healing, happiness, and love in the world.
Starting with you.

This book is dedicated to all of the sufferers of chronic pain and fatigue, whether from classic fibromyalgia or the many other conditions that are commonly misdiagnosed as fibromyalgia. Many of you have been mismanaged and even mistreated by the health-care system and by providers who generally have just not been informed enough about this disorder to provide you with a proper evaluation and treatment.

Some of you have even had your sincerity doubted; you have been told that your problems are all in your head and that there is nothing really wrong with you. If this has ever happened to you, it is unfortunate and inexcusable, and I am sorry. If this book helps even one of you who have had this kind of experience better understand what may really be wrong with you and find some solutions that help you feel better, if it helps you to be more empowered as an informed advocate for yourself as you try to navigate the health-care system going forward, then the effort will have been more than worth it.

CONTENTS

ACKNOWLEDGMENTS

First, I need to acknowledge the incredible work of my writing partner, Alison Rose Levy. Her ability to take my sometimes very complex ideas and former academic writings and presentations and wordsmith them into a form that everyone can understand and be entertained by is nothing short of astonishing. This book would simply not have been possible without her. The contributions of my good friend and colleague Ed McKiernan, DPT, who provided the movement and exercise instructions for the book based on his many years of physical therapy experience, and of Amy Berger, MS, who supplied the wonderful explanations of the relaxation techniques, made for a more comprehensive and better book, and for that I am most appreciative.

Much of what I have come to know about this mysterious thing we call fibromyalgia has been influenced over the past couple of decades by my friend and much respected colleague Michael J. Schneider, DC, PhD, a gifted doctor and researcher at the University of Pittsburgh School of Health and Rehabilitation Sciences. He has coauthored many pieces in medical journals and textbooks with me on fibromyalgia and has also been a true companion in this quest to shed some much-needed light on the subject for sufferers and health-care providers alike.

I need to thank my good friend Jonathan Lizotte, a true blessing in my life, for the "shove" that finally made this book happen. To all the colleagues and friends who have been incredibly supportive of my efforts—including everyone at Designs for Health, the University of Bridgeport, DrDavidBrady.com, and Whole-Body Medicine—I thank you. A special bit of gratitude is appropriate for one of my dearest friends,

Roger Koehler, for his unwavering encouragement, support, and guidance. Thanks to JJ Virgin and Drs. Amy Myers and William Davis for all of their valuable advice and for allowing me to learn from their experiences in the world of publishing.

I would be remiss to not acknowledge the privilege I have had to be represented by Celeste Fine and John Maas at Sterling Lord Literistic, Inc. and to be a writer for one of the absolute finest publishers in the health and wellness category, Rodale Inc. A special thanks to my editor at Rodale, Marisa Vigilante, who supported me and believed in the value of bringing this book to so many people who desperately need it.

I would like to thank my incredibly lovely wife, Stacey, for her support and understanding during all of time I spent with this project. I also would like to thank her for sharing all of her delicious and healthy recipes and for being the most spectacular and beautiful model I could have ever hoped for the instructional pictures in the movement and exercise sections of the book. Thanks also to my outstanding sons, Ian and Owen, for being so understanding when I missed more than a few of their hockey, baseball, and basketball games, and even a golf tournament or two, along the way. You could not have a prouder Daddy. I love you all, and you are why I do everything.

INTRODUCTION

Chronic pain affects nearly 100 million Americans, significantly more than diabetes, heart disease, and cancer combined, according to the Institute of Medicine. Ongoing fatigue affects an even greater number. This difficult combination of fatigue and body-wide chronic pain (often called fibromyalgia or FM) remains mysterious and confusing to many people and their doctors. A large study in the journal *Rheumatology* pointed out that referring physicians' and rheumatologists' initial diagnoses of fibromyalgia were accurate only 34 percent of the time. This means that an alarming 66 percent of those who were told by physicians that they had fibromyalgia were actually misdiagnosed.[1]

As a naturopathic medical doctor and nutritionist, I've found answers to unlock this puzzling group of interrelated illnesses, which I reveal in this comprehensive book, *The Fibro Fix*. For more than 23 years, I have treated thousands of patients seeking relief for what they considered a mystery illness—chronic global pain. And I have devised a protocol to help determine if, in fact, an individual is suffering from fibromyalgia—a nervous disorder involving the way the central nervous system processes pain—or from one of the several syndromes often misdiagnosed as fibromyalgia.

With a range of shared symptoms that often include achiness, pain, fatigue, brain fog, depression, sleep disturbance, and more, people labeled as suffering from fibromyalgia do not all have the same condition. As a result, they don't all respond to the same standard treatments. That is why understanding what *you* specifically experience is essential to recovery.

Because of the unique focus of my practice, I have been able to investigate fibromyalgia and global pain disorders, champion those who have them, and develop a pathway to diagnosis and treatment that can deliver you from pain for good.

My Background

People with this debilitating health challenge come from all over the country and the world to my practice, now in Fairfield, Connecticut. As a naturopathic medical physician (with initial training in physical medicine as a chiropractor), a functional medicine doctor, a board-certified clinical nutritionist, and a professor, my diverse background gives me a wide vantage point, one that few doctors possess, for getting to the bottom of pain syndromes.

That is why it's easier for me than it is for the average doctor to understand and differentiate the underlying biochemical and physical elements of these pain syndromes. In *The Fibro Fix*, I will pass that knowledge along to you.

In addition to my practice at Whole-Body Medicine in Fairfield, I also serve as the VP of the Division of Health Sciences and director of the Human Nutrition Institute at the University of Bridgeport in Connecticut. I am a prolific author of medical papers on fibromyalgia, and I have become one of the leading patient advocates in the field of fibromyalgia and global pain syndromes. I also wrote the book *Dr. Brady's Healthy Revolution*, which has helped thousands of people resolve their health issues. And I travel the world presenting at major conferences, teaching physicians and health-care providers, of many types, to learn the functional medicine approach that I use.

Initially, my practice grew by word of mouth from patients whom I had successfully treated. I had realized many years before that, by virtue of their training, doctors were ill-prepared to deal with this entity called fibromyalgia. While struggling to help these patients, I educated myself on this disorder. And after years of investigating the latest research, conferring with experts in the field, and working with colleagues who were also passionate about this topic, a clearer picture began to emerge for me.

What became clear is that the majority of doctors and other health-care providers knew very little about what this disorder really was—let alone how to effectively treat it. This led me to dedicate a part of my career to fibromyalgia research in order to better understand this nebulous condition, which has often been misdiagnosed and improperly treated. After years of sharing what I learned with my health-care colleagues, I decided to take the story right to the people who are directly affected—and since you are reading this book right now, that would be you!

Recently, my participation in several popular online health summits and programs has further increased my visibility, and this has drawn hundreds of new people to my clinical practice. My approach is well-recognized and highly regarded, leading to collaborations and presentations at major conferences with some of the health and wellness community's leading minds and advocates, including Drs. Mark Hyman, David Perlmutter, William Davis, Gerard Mullin, Amy Myers, Jeffrey Bland, Peter D'Adamo, Susan Blum, Kelly Brogan, Alan Christianson, and Izabella Wentz, as well as diet and fitness expert JJ Virgin.

Probing the Many Unanswered Questions

This book will delve into the true causes of your specific health problems. It will show you how to discover the precise conditions underlying your chronic pain and fatigue. And it will give you customized approaches to resolve these issues.

But why is it so hard to get help?

First off, just as many patients are confused about these syndromes, so are many physicians and other health-care professionals. I can't tell you how many people have told me that doctors they consulted discounted their complaints and flat-out told them that their problems were all in their head and that they should just take an antidepressant. I've even heard of doctors who eventually refused to continue seeing a patient with fibromyalgia syndrome. Unbelievable as this sounds, it's far too common for doctors—frustrated by their own inability to help—to abdicate their responsibility to find answers. Instead, they refer these patients to one specialist after another rather than working to get to the root cause of their patients' symptoms. While I sympathize with that frustration, it's a sad day when doctors, whose calling is to heal, give up.

But I understand why this happens. Fibromyalgia (FM) is extremely challenging to diagnose. There is no single lab test doctors can do, and they must rely on patients' reports of their symptoms. Without the clear grasp of this illness that this book offers, both patients and their doctors are often confused. To add to the difficulty, many other diseases and problems can mask themselves as fibromyalgia, leading both doctor and patient down many blind alleys. Without a deeper understanding of fibromyalgia, arriving at an accurate diagnosis may take many years. Some people actually welcome a lab report with a definitive finding that they have a serious disease, so that they finally know what the problem is. To understand why FM and associated syndromes have fallen into this black hole, let's take a few steps back and look at the overall health-care environment.

The Current State of Health Care in America

Along with the millions of people suffering from various forms of chronic disease, FM sufferers fall into a poorly acknowledged gap in our health-care system. In many ways, the old models of medicine no longer work—particularly in addressing the chronic degenerative disorders of our time: diabetes, obesity, autoimmune diseases, high blood pressure, osteoarthritis, chronic fatigue, and fibromyalgia, to name a few. As chronic disease rates mount with every passing year, people are less and less satisfied with the limited therapeutic options available from conventional medicine.

Chronic Diseases: What Are They?

The US Centers for Disease Control and Prevention (CDC) and the Partnership to Fight Chronic Disease define chronic diseases as "ongoing, generally incurable illnesses or conditions, such as heart disease, asthma, cancer, and diabetes."[2] The CDC acknowledges that these diseases can often be prevented, or managed through early detection, improved diet, exercise, and treatment. Yet, chronic diseases are the leading cause of death and disability in the United States. It is estimated that 149 million Americans in 2015 (nearly 48 percent of the population) have at least one chronic disease. And seven out of every 10 deaths in the

United States are the result of chronic illnesses, which kill more than 1.7 million Americans annually.[3] Figure I.1 shows the increasing toll chronic disease is taking in the United States.

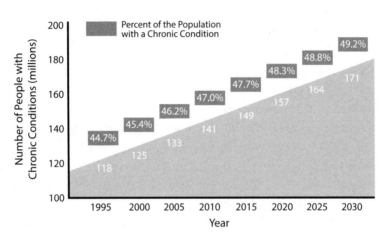

FIGURE I.1 PERCENTAGE OF THE US POPULATION WITH A CHRONIC CONDITION

Source: S. Y. Wu and A. Green, Projection of Chronic Illness Prevalence and Cost Inflation, RAND Corporation, October 2000.

While there are specific treatments for cancer (chemotherapy, radiation, and surgery), heart disease (statin medications, stents, and bypass surgery), and other common lethal diseases, these treatments are costly, uncomfortable, and not always entirely effective. Sadly, more and more people are learning from tough personal experiences that medicine doesn't always deliver on its promises.

Medicine's Promise

To understand why conventional medicine is not doing a better job of delivering health, both for FM and many other health problems, let's take a closer look at one of conventional medicine's key promises: increased life expectancy. Is modern medicine delivering on that prediction? Unfortunately, not.

Increases in the average human life span have fallen far short of oft-repeated predictions. In fact, the big leaps in life expectancy that we base our hopes upon mainly occurred back in the first half of the twentieth century. And these, by and large, were not due to costly and advanced medical procedures or modern drugs. They were due to better public health conditions and the use of antibiotic medications to treat acute bacterial infections.

Over the last several decades, increases in life span have been steady but minimal—and nowhere near the level that was predicted decades ago. Back in my training days, my medical mentors thought that by 2015 people would routinely live to 100, 110, or even 120 years of age. Despite the tantalizing lure of novel treatments and magical breakthroughs, the promise to extend longevity has not materialized yet.

According to a survey by the Pew Research Center, "many Americans do not look happily on the prospect of living much longer lives. They see peril as well as promise in biomedical advances, and more think it would be a bad thing than a good thing for society if people lived decades longer than is possible today."[4]

Why? Because they believe that radically longer life spans would strain the country's resources and would only be available to the wealthy.

Now, with the epidemic of overweight and obesity, and all the ensuing health issues, we actually face the prospect of the first American generation that is predicted to live a shorter life span than their parent's generation.

What lies behind the ballyhooed promises of longevity? Advanced modern medicine, despite all of the dramatic examples of heroic life-saving interventions for acute disorders and trauma, has delivered too little in return for its massive costs. When you look at where most of our health-care dollars actually go, the reality is that they are spent giving the elderly a few more months of life. And given the disabilities and maladies that can come with growing old, it's often a few more months with a poor quality of life—not something most people want.

A Choice

To give you a better idea of what I am talking about, consider this hypothetical scenario. Suppose you could choose better health, find freedom from global pain, enjoy plentiful energy, sleep soundly and easily, and live until the age of 86. If you happened to be 40 years old right now, then you would have good health beginning today and for the next 46 years. Your other choice: You don't enjoy health and vitality, but when you approach the end of your life, you get to prolong it for 3 to 6 months—no matter the state of your mental or physical health.

Let me unequivocally state that as both a doctor and a human being, I value all life, even life at its end for those in poor health. What I am inviting you to contemplate is what *you* would actually prefer given the choice. Of course, the reality is that today the current health-care-management system makes the choice for us. And it chooses medical procedures at the end of life. Very few health-care expenditures are devoted to preventing the diseases that often kill us, even though these interventions are far cheaper than the costly medical procedures done in the final months of life. This bias in health care is reinforced by the way health insurance is currently structured; it is difficult to get coverage for anything preventive that might fall into the "alternative health" category.

A False Measurement

But more and more people—including those who suffer from global pain syndromes—are discovering, as you will in this book, that there's another choice, and they are learning how to access it.

By understanding the difference between the two choices, you can more readily grasp why health advocates now suggest that the way we measure health is faulty. Instead of looking at marginal increases in life span across the population, often accounted for by a few months of prolonged life in the elderly, we should aim toward reducing disability and suffering over the entire life span.

How can we change health care so that it really delivers? Is it even possible to change our health-care system to better serve our health and wellness needs? What is standard medicine overlooking? When people encounter FM or any other disorder that is not properly resolved by the methods of the conventional medical system, they begin asking questions. By looking at your overall health and wellness more holistically, I hope to help you understand why it has been so hard up until now to get answers and solutions for your global pain syndrome, whether it's FM or another problem.

Why Crisis-Oriented Health Does Not Relieve Chronic Complaints

If I had to point out the single biggest flaw in the standard medical approach, it's this: Our health-care system has little to offer until health problems are severe, necessitating crisis management. Obviously, there's a great need for crisis care, but what about identifying and intervening before health problems become critical or life threatening? In reality, the current system is a "disease care" system, not a "health-care" system. When doctors and other health-care professionals get involved only after problems have emerged, people face an uphill battle recovering from a *presenting* illness, when it would have been far easier to *prevent* that illness. However, make no mistake about it, this approach makes the health-care industry a lot of money.

As a doctor myself, I recommend high-tech medicine for its great treatments in crisis situations, such as traumatic injuries, acute infectious diseases, and critical care. However, despite the staggering amount of money being spent on crisis-centered medicine, these approaches don't work well for the majority of illnesses that debilitate the population, weaken health, and shorten lives. If you have FM or another global pain syndrome, along with millions of other Americans, you live with the poor outcomes that result from the standard medical paradigm.

Remember the question I posed about living a healthier life throughout your life span? In this book, I contend that we must deploy treatments that make that possible. I don't believe that as a society we can afford to rely solely on medical approaches that can treat injuries incurred in a car accident but overlook the major health problems suffered by millions of people. Because most doctors were never trained in, and haven't taken the time to look into, the extensive body of research supporting the use of the many proven-effective lifestyle changes I will offer in this book, they denigrate them and try to suppress their use. These include stress reduction practices, dietary changes, and the specific and smart use of nutritional supplements, nutraceuticals, botanical medicines, and other preventive approaches. The sad result is that people miss out on the opportunity to maintain health and protect themselves from disease.

Fibromyalgia is one of many chronic, life-debilitating ailments that fall by the wayside, or are poorly managed, when we neglect ways to build and enhance overall health and wellness and increase vibrancy.

A Change Is Coming

Fortunately, things are beginning to change—and my approach to treating global pain is part of that shift. Although conventional doctors have been standoffish toward the array of available tools for health promotion, more and more people, and their doctors, are trying them. Whether experiencing health challenges like FM or taking care of loved ones suffering from chronic disease, people are less and less willing to sit back and suffer, hoping their doctors will eventually find something to help them. I applaud and thank all of you who want to take matters into your own hands. You and others like you are participating in the meteoric rise of integrative and complementary approaches to manage chronic disorders and more aggressively prevent disease in the first place. In response to the growing need and interest, many clinicians and researchers have continued to study and develop the most effective approaches. Today, basic tools to lose weight, manage stress, and prevent illness are much more well known, even by the general public, than they were when I first trained and entered practice.

But when it comes to some of the more complex chronic disorders, people are still often stymied and overly reliant on doctors, many of whom, for the reasons I've mentioned, don't understand the interlocking pain syndromes covered in this book. What you and other global pain and fatigue sufferers need is a way to access the emerging body of knowledge about health *now*. And that is what you'll get in the coming pages of *The Fibro Fix*.

The New Medicine

Some of you may already be familiar with the new health model this book is based on. Over the last four decades, many concerned health-care professionals, scientists, and researchers have been asking the very same questions I pose in this chapter, and they are coming up with new answers. This new breed of doctors is changing how medicine approaches and treats illness. As one of those who are participating in this growing trend, let me clear up some confusion, since it's referred to by many names: I prefer the term *functional* medicine, because this new model looks at how well various systems of your body are functioning and finds ways to make them work better.[5] But it is also referred to as *metabolic* medicine, *comprehensive* medicine, *complementary* medicine, and *integrative* medicine. By any name, however, this movement is growing within the scientific-based health-care community—which includes medical, naturopathic, osteopathic, and chiropractic doctors, as well as many other clinicians, such as nutritionists, nurse practicioners, acupuncturists, health coaches, and many more.

I have been a participant in this movement almost since its inception well over 20 years ago. The advice I offer you here is based on both my own clinical experience and a body of clinical wisdom and research developed by this new breed of doctors, researchers, and clinicians over several decades. An added bonus is that wherever you live, you can access some of the more advanced tests and recommendations in *The Fibro Fix* if you need them. In the Additional Resources section (page 259) and on FibroFix.com, I will also offer ways to find practitioners who can implement my recommendations.

While there used to be a rigid demarcation between conventional and functional practice, this is changing, too. Many of the health-care providers who felt uncomfortable with approaches dubbed "alternative" are now singing a new tune. There is significant interest from many nationally renowned physicians in the hallowed ivy-covered towers and halls of academic orthodox medicine. The reasons for this are many, but leading the list is the fact that it makes so much sense. This new medicine packages this emerging paradigm into a scientifically valid, research-based body of knowledge and possesses a level of credibility no alternative approach has ever before enjoyed.

Functional Medicine

Thousands of conventionally trained physicians and other health-care providers have migrated to this model despite continued criticism by the orthodox medical establishment. However, the 2014 opening of centers for functional and integrative medicine at the Cleveland Clinic Foundation and George Washington University are a testament to the growth of this approach. With this new model, the focus is now on optimal function rather than the presence, or absence, of disease. Let's take a closer look at how it works.

Functional medicine is patient-centered, science-based health care that identifies and addresses underlying biochemical, physiological, environmental, and psychological factors in order to reverse the progression of disease and enhance vitality. According to the Institute for Functional Medicine (functionalmedicine.org), "functional medicine is a personalized, systems-oriented model that empowers patients and practitioners to achieve the highest expression of health by working in collaboration to address the underlying causes of disease."[6]

In his book *Healing the Hyper Active Brain Through the New Science of Functional Medicine*, Michael R. Lyon, MD, examines what is unique about this approach.

> Most medical treatments are considered satisfactory if they simply reduce or eliminate the symptoms of a disease, or even just alter the results of a laboratory test. In many instances, little consideration is given for the overall quality of a patient's life or ability to function as a productive member of society.[7]

Dr. Lyon also notes, "Rather than depending solely on single, powerful treatments such as drugs or surgery, functional medicine relies more upon intelligent and individualized combinations of treatments or protocols."[8] In order to be consistent with functional-medicine principles, Dr. Lyon says a treatment should:

1. Have little or no risk of doing harm and be as free as possible of unpleasant side effects

2. Improve symptoms and overall function, as well as quality of life

3. Help correct the underlying cause or causes of the disorder

4. Improve the long-term outlook for the patient

In *The Fibro Fix*, I bring just this kind of approach to FM and its often-misdiagnosed associated syndromes.

Obviously, conventional medical approaches are necessary for treating acute illness, trauma, and end-stage disease and in fact excel in these circumstances. However, chronically ill patients, like those suffering from global pain and fatigue syndromes, can't seem to get an accurate or definitive medical diagnosis from their standard medical providers. Because the functional approach is so successful with chronic ailments like FM, many people are working with (and in some measure helping to educate) their conventional providers. In other cases, patients are moving on to consult with this new type of physician. If now, or later, you feel the need to consult with a new doctor versed in the approach I offer in *The Fibro Fix*, I advise that you look for one who will work *with* you in managing your treatment and who blends complementary and conventional approaches based on your individual situation.

To successfully implement this approach, the doctor will need a strong working knowledge of diet, vitamins, minerals, herbs, stress-management techniques, and other therapeutic interventions in addition to drugs and surgery, since this program depends on nontoxic and noninvasive interventions whenever possible. Many doctors are intrigued but intimidated by this approach because they lack training in these matters and don't have the time or the resources to learn about it. This book contains excellent information for doctors, as well.

Digging into the Research

Based on this new model, I set out to unravel the mystery of fibromyalgia and soon found a kindred spirit in Michael J. Schneider, DC, PhD. Now a researcher at the University of Pittsburgh School of Health and Rehabilitation Sciences, Dr. Schneider originally trained as a chiropractic doctor and later specialized in myofascial therapy before pursuing his PhD and researching approaches to chronic global pain in the field of integrative medicine.

Over 15 years ago, Dr. Schneider and I decided to collaborate. In order to find answers and educate our physician colleagues, we conducted detailed systematic research reviews and published our findings and hypotheses about fibromyalgia in medical journals, professional publications, and medical textbooks. We also offered countless lectures to professional audiences around the country and the world. And we contributed to articles and books aimed at the general public, hoping to reach people diagnosed, either correctly or incorrectly, with FM.

Out of this work, we developed a simplified and logical framework for determining if people really had a global pain syndrome, such as classic fibromyalgia, or if other issues were causing their problems. You'll access that very same framework in this book. Because of our good results in resolving symptoms once considered "too complicated" to figure out, other doctors started referring patients with these kinds of problems to us.

Since those early years, I've now had decades of solid success resolving FM and related chronic global pain syndromes based on this approach. My many years of clinical work and research have transformed me into a passionate advocate for patients labeled with FM as well as for all those who suffer from misdiagnosed associated syndromes and disorders. My goal in *The Fibro Fix* is to offer you a baseline program that provides initial relief and information that can lead to the treatments that will bring you real and lasting results. For me, personally, there is nothing more satisfying than knowing that I have helped many patients finally find the solution to their pain and fatigue, often after many years of searching.

How to Use This Book

Here's a brief overview of how this book works. First, I recommend that you immediately begin following my 21-day Fibro-Fix Foundational Plan. It begins with these simple steps to feel better fast—detox, diet, relaxation, and movement. As you begin to use the recipes, shakes, exercise plans, supplement information, and stress-management techniques, you will reduce inflammation, eliminate food allergens and sensitivities, address low energy, and begin moving safely once again. While this plan is not a cure for fibromyalgia—or any other disorder erroneously labeled as fibromyalgia—it will help you restore a healthy baseline and begin to alleviate symptoms. This first-step foundational intervention will start the process of rejuvenating your metabolism while you continue to read the book and learn more about what may be actually causing your unique problems.

From there, this book will go on to clarify the specifics of your syndrome, its causes, and the treatments that can address them once and for all.

Many doctors fail to recognize that each individual with pain and fatigue is unique. The assumption that all pain sufferers have the same disease due to the same causes is just plain wrong. Although the very different pain syndromes I cover are mistakenly placed into one big bucket, there are several different categories of ailments that can produce similar symptoms. And unless your illness is placed in the right bucket, the recommended treatments are unlikely to work for you. In fact, they may worsen the disorder or trigger undesirable side effects or symptoms. The good news is that by reading (and taking the assessments within) the book's first three chapters, you'll find the right bucket, the one that corresponds to the kind of disorder you suffer from. You'll then get great help from the chapter(s) that apply to you. By following the right recommendations, you'll very likely join the 80 percent of global pain sufferers who have followed my program to significant and often permanent relief. Why not 100 percent? There is always a percentage of people who, for one reason or another, do not respond to intervention— whether it's due to major ongoing stress in their lives, poor diet, or other medical issues.

While I will offer guidance on the proper use of medications when needed, I differ from the majority of doctors who are quick to prescribe painkillers and antidepressants. Instead, throughout this book, I will show you why taking a more comprehensive, individualized, and holistic approach is what you need to make a real difference. *The Fibro Fix* holds the key to solving chronic global pain and fatigue so that you can regain your strength, energy, and hope for a pain-free and energetic future.

So please join me on a journey to find that pain-free, vibrant, and energetic person that you and your loved ones have been missing.

CHAPTER 1

FIBROMYALGIA AND CHRONIC GLOBAL PAIN SYNDROMES— CLEARING UP THE CONFUSION

I decided to write this book in response to the mass confusion over fibromyalgia and the associated syndromes incorrectly diagnosed as fibromyalgia. Together, these syndromes afflict literally millions of Americans.[1] For decades, too many have suffered in silence from these illnesses because medicine has been slow to understand them—and slower still to offer the right diagnoses and specific treatments. Sadly, there are millions of people who fit one of the following categories.

- People who have been diagnosed with fibromyalgia but still have questions about their condition

- People who are being treated for fibromyalgia but aren't feeling better yet and wonder if something else might be wrong

- People who have been told that they have fibromyalgia but have been misdiagnosed and may be suffering from another illness

- People who are still struggling to identify what is wrong with them, even though they've been to countless doctors

The bottom line is that those who experience fibromyalgia and other chronic global pain syndromes are one of the most substantial—and underserved—segments of pain sufferers. If you suffer from global pain, I feel for you. I am writing *The Fibro Fix* because, after working with so many patients who have struggled with global pain, I know your struggle. In fact, my mother-in-law was once a sufferer until I married her daughter and helped fix her fibromyalgia!

My approach begins with understanding the complexity of this inter-related cluster of illnesses, which—for now—I discuss under the broad term *fibromyalgia syndrome,* or FM. This is the foundation for finding and implementing new and more effective treatments. The first step is to determine precisely what you are experiencing, and the second is to identify what is causing your specific complaints. Surprisingly, standard health care often fails to explore those two simple steps.

In this book, my goal is to help you understand why it has been so hard until now to get answers and solutions for your pain. FM is myste-rious because each case is individual, and without an individualized approach, people and their doctors can't readily arrive at the right treat-ments. Unfortunately, the US health care system is not yet ready to accommodate individualized treatment—even though that is what is required to help you resolve your pain. Later in this chapter, and throughout the book, I will examine the factors in our health-care sys-tem that make it unnecessarily challenging for patients with FM. You need to fully grasp this in order to move forward, put past hardships behind you, and be ready for all the benefits you'll get from this new approach.

I want you to feel those benefits right away. So, as soon as you read this chapter—or for that matter, *as you read it*—I invite you to undertake my 21-day foundational program, which you'll find in Chapter 2. By fol-lowing just three simple steps you'll begin to alleviate your symptoms at once, whatever their underlying cause may be. You'll automatically revive low energy; reduce any inflammation that may be driving your pain; eliminate food allergens and sensitivities, which can also cause inflam-mation; reduce your stress; and start to regain critical mobility. As you follow the plan, go on to read Chapter 3, where I explain that along with fibromyalgia, we need to look at additional kinds of health problems that *aren't* fibromyalgia—but are often misdiagnosed as such. Both fibromyalgia and each kind of FM mimic require their own specific treatment, which I discuss in Chapters 4, 5, and 6. Understanding the distinctions among classic fibromyalgia and its imitators is half the battle. You'll also take a test to help you determine if there's a likelihood that your issue *is* classic fibromyalgia.

In Chapter 7, I will troubleshoot additional and more advanced treatments, tests, and options, should these be necessary, as determined by your progress through the program. And in Chapter 8, I present a maintenance plan for going forward as your health improves.

This book will ensure that you have all the resources you need to get to the bottom of your chronic pain syndrome and regain your health.

Who Suffers from Fibromyalgia Syndrome?

About 15 million people in the United States and about 20 million in the rest of the world are suffering from FM, according to a 2011 National Institutes of Health finding. And that figure may be even higher, for several reasons. A prime reason, as you'll hear me say over and over again, is that fibromyalgia is notoriously hard to diagnose; you'll learn from reading this book that it's often mistaken for illnesses with strikingly similar symptoms. Another reason the statistics may be skewed is that men and women tend to perceive pain differently, and as a group, women have been shown in research to perceive pain at lower pressure thresholds when it is applied to their soft tissues than men.[2]

THE COSTS OF FIBROMYALGIA

Fibromyalgia costs a lot of money—both to patients and to society. A 2014 study found that 34 percent of fibromyalgia sufferers spend from $100 to $1,000 per month over and above their insurance on health professionals. In addition there's lost work time. Researchers estimate that fibromyalgia is responsible for a 1 to 2 percent loss in the nation's overall productivity. And failure to diagnose FM correctly has its own costs, in doctor visits, prescriptions, lab tests, and lost time.[3]

Based on the statistics we have, although fibromyalgia strikes both genders and all races, it generally strikes people between the ages of 20 and 55 and affects women about ten times more than men. The typical fibromyalgia sufferer is a Caucasian woman. But since white women are also the segment of the public most likely to schedule an office visit when they experience a health problem, it's possible that is skewing the statistics somewhat.[4]

Although a precise cause is not known, classic fibromyalgia is a disorder of the central nervous system—in effect, a wiring problem—that may be triggered by trauma or early psychological issues. While environmental factors play a role, there is very likely a genetic component, as well: Up to 28 percent of children born to a parent with fibromyalgia develop it themselves.[5]

Symptoms of Fibromyalgia

While there may be many other possible symptoms of FM, let's start with the most common one: pain. The pain of true, or classic, fibromyalgia is referred to as global, affecting the upper and lower extremities on both sides of the body as well the torso. This type of pain is not just in one region, or even several regions, of the body—for example the shoulder, lower back, and pelvis. Global pain is experienced all over the body.

Do You Have Global Pain or Regional Pain?

The pain diagrams filled out by patients in Figure 1.1 illustrate the difference between global pain and regional pain.

It's actually quite easy to distinguish global pain from localized or regional pain. Suppose you accidentally hit your finger with a hammer. It will hurt like crazy! Doctors call this localized pain since it's confined to a specific area that you can readily pinpoint. The pain also comes from a clearly known cause—in this case, the hammer. In contrast, global pain is not limited to any particular area of the body. The pain you feel is widespread. It involves your arms and legs on both sides of the body and is usually felt in your torso, as well. There is acute sensitivity to touch and sometimes light and sound. Even mild stimuli, like a pat on the back,

FIGURE 1.1 GLOBAL PAIN VERSUS REGIONAL PAIN

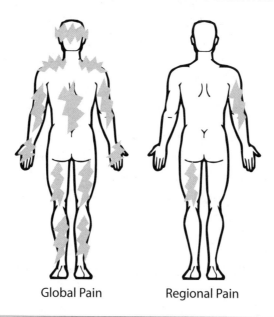

Global Pain   Regional Pain

may feel painful. But while the pain is real, the source of the pain seems like a mystery; this is one keynote of chronic global pain syndromes.

Other Common Symptoms

Global pain is usually accompanied by other symptoms, like extreme fatigue, depression, brain fog, and irritable bowel syndrome (IBS). A troublesome standalone disorder in itself, IBS often accompanies true fibromyalgia and may include intestinal cramping, bloating, gassiness, diarrhea, and/or constipation. This broad range of potential symptoms makes fibromyalgia and other associated chronic pain syndromes that can masquerade as FM hard to diagnose.

I wish I could tell you that there's one single test that your doctor can use to confirm a diagnosis. Unfortunately, there's not. There's no fibromyalgia box that you can check off on a lab report request. Yes, there are test results that are highly correlated with fibromyalgia. But the reality is that to arrive at an accurate diagnosis it requires first *ruling out* other illnesses. All of this makes it very difficult for both you and your health-care providers. If you're suffering from chronic global pain, it's hard enough to function at all, let alone run around looking for the rare doctor who knows how to figure out what's wrong with you.[6]

That is why I wrote this book—to help you navigate your symptoms and start to heal.

Why Is FM So Tough to Deal With?

Fibromyalgia syndrome is not merely difficult for the people who suffer from it. It's also hard on their relationships and families. As time drags on, with no remedy or relief, with the raised and dashed hopes of finding a doctor who can help, the families, colleagues, and friends of fibro-

---

WHAT FM SUFFERERS MAY EXPERIENCE

Deep muscular aches and pains. You may experience deep muscular aches—especially in the most used muscle groups, such as the large muscles of the legs, pelvis, upper shoulders, and arms—along with throbbing, shooting, or stabbing pain.

Burning. You may feel intense burning sensations in these areas, as well.

Exhaustion. You may feel as though your arms and legs are weighed down by concrete blocks, and your body may be so drained of energy that every task requires great effort.

Sleeplessness. You may experience various forms of sleeplessness, such as discomfort or active pain that keeps you awake or wakes you up, the inability to go to sleep, waking up too early and not getting back to sleep, or sleeping and waking up feeling groggy and unrefreshed.

Acute sensitivity to stimuli. You may be extremely sensitive to touch, light, or sound.

Depression. You may experience a sadness with no clear-cut cause, a loss of pleasure in enjoyable activities, feelings of guilt and worthlessness, a wish for death, and weight loss or gain due to emotional eating.

---

myalgia sufferers may themselves begin to doubt whether their loved one's or friend's pain and other symptoms are really real. Many people have aches and pains, especially as they age. So how do you validate the difference between more routine complaints and global chronic pain syndromes?

This becomes more challenging when, from the outset, there's a common bias that people experiencing pain are whiners or complainers who should just grin and bear it. Men in particular are more likely to hold such mistaken attitudes. These unhelpful beliefs were reinforced for many decades by the medical profession. For example, in the 1950s, doctors classified fibromyalgia as psychogenic rheumatism, a form of rheumatism originating in the mind. Translated, this would mean that the arthritis, or joint pain, is somehow imaginary. But this was wrong on

Skin changes. You may have swelling, and your skin may become blotchy, shiny, blue, or have itchy red bumps similar to hives.

Abnormal sweating. You may experience abnormal sweating.

Brain fog. You may also suffer from brain fog, a condition in which you have trouble concentrating, finding words, or retaining new information, with the density of the fog corresponding to the severity of your pain.

Joint stiffness. You may perceive stiffness in your joints, especially in the morning.

Headaches. Recurrent tension headaches or migraines are present in 50 to 70 percent of fibromyalgia sufferers. The symptoms can be severe, can occur one or two times per week, and can be accompanied by a migraine.

Balance issues. You may have trouble balancing, which can affect your walking and increase your chances of falling.

Digestive disorders. A large percentage of FM sufferers have gut issues, such as constipation, diarrhea, abdominal pain, gas and bloating, irritable bowel syndrome, nausea, acid reflux, or slowed digestion.

both counts—FM isn't a form of rheumatism, and it isn't imaginary.

When people who suffer from global pain do finally manage to begin the all-too-often extended process of dragging their exhausted bodies around to doctors, instead of getting the help they need, they often encounter misdiagnosis or end up with prescriptions for drugs that do little to improve their condition, and may even worsen it.

Ultimately, many FM sufferers turn to mental-health professionals to help them manage the depression, anxiety, and social isolation that result from living for years with an illness that many people doubt is genuine, that doctors can't identify, and for which they believed there was no real answer. But there are answers, and the whole aim of *The Fibro Fix* is to offer you the ones exactly right for your condition.

Why Most Doctors Can't Help

"I've seen fibromyalgia patients who have pain all over and doctors have said, 'Well you have this type of neck pain, you have elbow pain, and you have knee pain,'" reports Robert Bonakdar, MD, director of pain management at the Scripps Center for Integrative Medicine in San Diego. "Patients then see different specialists, but no one puts the pieces together."[7]

Initially, I too felt this same perplexity. In taking medical histories in the early years of treating people with fibromyalgia, I was frankly shocked to learn how often these folks, suffering with pain and other challenges, were discounted, misdiagnosed, and even mistreated by their doctors. At the outset, I felt less than totally convinced that what I had been taught during my clinical training would help me help them. Were the conventional medical approaches, like pain and antidepressant medications, effective in treating this disorder? Were common alternative and complementary approaches—like chiropractic manipulation, acupuncture, and massage—effective? I began to discover that while sometimes they were, often they were not.[8]

Along with the dawning awareness that our simplistic approaches didn't deliver real relief, I was in for another surprise: Many, if not most, of my colleagues, despite their limited success and incomplete knowledge of this disease, were convinced that they understood fibromyalgia and were offering their patients the right treatments. It's as if health-care professionals themselves were in a kind of brain fog, confused by the vast array of symptoms and their possible causes. As my doubts about the approach *du jour* collided with my colleagues' misplaced certainties, I began to realize that we were all stumbling in the dark without a flashlight. The only difference was that I knew it and they, it seemed to me, did not. So I began to search for a flashlight, for the understanding that would shed light on the true nature of fibromyalgia and how to treat it.

The Quest for an Answer

After undertaking an extensive study of FM, including an exhaustive review of the medical literature and research studies, and reaching out to some of the leading experts in the field for guidance and opinions, I started to understand the complexity of this illness and how important it is to systematically determine what a patient is actually experiencing and what is causing the specific complaints of achiness, pain, fatigue, brain fog, depression, sleep disturbance, and more. It was very apparent to me that since not all of my patients were responsive to the same treatments, they were not all suffering from the same illness.[9]

For example, Diane, a 60-year-old patient of mine, who was ultimately found to have fibromyalgia, received five different diagnoses over a 3-year period. In rapid succession, she was told she had Raynaud's phenomenon, rheumatoid arthritis, gout, depression, and arteriosclerosis. But though she was suffering from *all* of these conditions except Raynaud's phenomenon, everyone had missed the fibromyalgia.

Conversely, there are cases where patients are thought to have fibromyalgia but are actually suffering from other illnesses. For example, Joan, a physical therapist colleague of mine, noticed that Emily, a woman in her midthirties who had been diagnosed with fibromyalgia, didn't fully fit the profile. Joan recommended that Emily see a neurologist. After a number of diagnostic tests, the neurologist found that Emily's symptoms were related to her use of the antidepressant citalopram. Side effects of citalopram include somnolence (sleepiness), insomnia, and anxiety. As you can see, even a correctly prescribed medication can be the culprit in the sudden appearance of symptoms.

Unfortunately, the average physician may not be able to troubleshoot all the factors that must be examined to get to the bottom of this disorder. To become comfortable with the approach I offer my patients—and will provide in this book—mainstream doctors often must forget a great deal of their medical training. Although intuitively obvious to the average person, my program does not follow the way modern physicians are generally trained to think.

The Stigma of Global Pain Disorders

Because fibromyalgia is so poorly understood and the causes of fibromyalgia and syndromes mislabeled as FM often remain invisible, doctors will frequently try to "manage" the patient by keeping her at arm's length. Along with ordinary folks, some health-care providers may secretly think that fibromyalgia sufferers are hypochondriacs or neurotics who are faking their symptoms to get sympathy. People who believe in toughing it out may privately feel critical of those who don't seem to be able to live by that ethos. After months and years of this kind of doubt, even if no one expresses disbelief about the illness out loud, FM sufferers pick up on it. Remember, this is a condition of heightened sensitivity, even oversensitivity. Although much of this heightened sensitivity is tactile and sensate, some people also experience heightened emotional sensitivity. As a result, they may wind up feeling ashamed or guilty. Janet (name changed), a recovered patient of mine, shared this with me, and I share it with you because it describes the feelings of self-blame that plague many sufferers.

> There is a lot of guilt with this disease. Most days, by the time my husband gets home from work, I am in bed. It's humiliating to try to tell him how I have to stop doing my own work and sleep for the rest of the afternoon. Even though he is very sympathetic, I still feel that it's my fault—and his kindness only makes me feel worse, because behind it I see the frustration, anger, and blame that he can't talk about. I even feel guilt toward our cats, since I never play with them anymore. And I feel ashamed that I am relying on antidepressants to keep me going, even though they're really not working so well.

It's Not Your Fault

If you are suffering from long-standing pain and fatigue, the first thing to know is that it's not your fault. Whether it's truly fibromyalgia or one of the illnesses that mimic its symptoms (which you'll learn about in this book), your problems are all too real, despite what many people think. The issue is not patients who are faking their symptoms but widespread misinformation—misinformation that is confusing patients and doctors alike.

For example, it's no news flash that pain-killing medications, which doctors routinely prescribe for global pain disorders, are quite likely to make you feel groggy and foggy—common complaints of people with FM and associated symptoms. Antidepressants and sleep medications often have the same effect. This is just one simple example of how failing to get to the root cause compounds rather than relieves symptoms. Sufferers don't know whether their grogginess is due to FM or to medication—and it could be either or both.

Bottom line? Relieving pain by *addressing the cause* of the pain—so that the pain goes away, period—is not the same as dulling the pain. I am emphasizing this distinction so that you can grasp what this book offers and why you haven't readily found this type of solution before. That positive outcome may seem hard to imagine for people who have struggled for years with global pain and fatigue syndromes, yet in close collaboration with my patients, and using the right diagnostic approach, I have been able to resolve their pain and other symptoms time and time again. Obviously, there are no guarantees, but I am confident because I've seen it happen so often.

Carol's Story

Carol, a woman in her late thirties debilitated by her symptoms of global pain, fatigue, brain fog, and irritable bowel syndrome, came into my office. She couldn't hold a job and had moved back home with her mother. Carol had been through the typical mill, going first to her primary care doctor, who sent her to a rheumatologist. She then went on to consult with an orthopedist, a physical therapist, and a mental-health counselor, looking for relief.

Despite all of this disjointed care, no one had taken responsibility for managing her case. By the time Carol came to see me, she was on 13 medications—six to manage specific symptoms like depression, pain, muscle spasm, and constipation and seven to counteract the side effects of the first six. For example, she was on an antinausea medication to counteract a side effect of the pain medication. All of this on top of suffering from a chronic illness.

The first thing I recommended was for Carol to start on an anti-inflammatory, antiallergy/sensitivity diet and to follow a detox program for several weeks, the same ones you'll do in the next chapter. With her energy improved and her pain lessened, it soon became possible to reduce and eventually eliminate some of the unnecessary medications she took.

Since Carol was not having muscle spasms, it was a no-brainer to stop the muscle relaxant. Since neither the anti-inflammatory nor the pain reliever was working, we decided she could stop taking those, too. I recommended specific nutritional supplements, and Carol noticed an increase in her energy right away. In addition, I prescribed physical treatments, which included massage, relaxation exercises, and stretching. Following 4 months of intense treatment, she got off all of her medications.

Six months after Carol first walked into my office, she came in for her appointment, and my receptionist thought she was a new patient and asked for her name. Instead of being beaten down by a chronic illness, Carol was outgoing and upbeat. She had even signed a lease on a new apartment.

Like many FM sufferers, Carol had gone through a difficult childhood and had been abused in prior romantic relationships. Because of these experiences, she came to feel as though she must always be prepared for disaster. Thinking back on her life, she could rarely recall a time when she had felt protected. Although it may surprise those unfamiliar with FM, Carol's childhood experience is just one of the hundreds of examples I've seen of a tense, stress-ridden, and unsafe environment in early life. Often there has been verbal and even physical abuse from a parent, usually the father. When such experiences take place while the nervous system is developing, it's not surprising that they can produce a life-long impact, setting up a predisposition to global pain syndromes and IBS. Sadly, when these FM sufferers enter the medical system, seeking help, the pattern is often replicated when doctors with an inadequate grasp of this syndrome dismiss their complaints.

Medical Misdiagnosis of FM

For over two decades, the health-insurance industry defined fibromyalgia syndrome as generalized pain that isn't associated with any injury. But this "kitchen sink" definition was too broad, and as a result, plenty of people were—and are—receiving prescriptions for painkillers or antidepressants, when these drugs do nothing to address the underlying causes of their illness and, in some cases, may even worsen it.

In 1990, the American College of Rheumatology (ACR) developed the first diagnostic criteria for FM, using a scoring system based on a physical examination by a doctor. To qualify for a diagnosis of fibromyalgia, the patient had to have a minimum of 11 out of 18 anatomical areas that were tender to moderate pressure as well as pain above and below the waist on both sides of the body, along the torso, and in the extremities.[10]

That sounds good unless you probe into the history and discover that these criteria were never really meant to be used by practicing doctors to diagnose patients. They were meant for use by researchers studying FM—an entirely different matter.

However, given doctors' desperation for any diagnostic tool, these criteria fell into common use and resulted in significant overdiagnosis of FM. One problem was that this tool didn't adequately discriminate between true, or classic, FM and other disorders that, as you will see, met the criteria's standards.

The ACR revised the criteria in 2010 and again in 2011. The current criteria consist of a Widespread Pain Index, based on a patient's own report of pain, and a symptom severity index, calculated from a patient's responses to a questionnaire. Questions deal with the presence of symptoms such as fatigue, sleep disturbance, cognitive deficit, inability to concentrate, anxiety, and depression. The symptoms must be present for at least 3 months and must not be attributable to any other disorder. (You'll be asked to take a similar questionnaire in Chapter 3.)

Although the revised ACR criteria are somewhat improved, they now do not require the doctor to actually touch and examine the patient. Instead, the diagnosis relies solely on the patient's report of pain in various parts of the body. Yet a hands-on exam is crucial to determining whether pain is global or localized. Sadly, after many years of relying on CAT scans, MRIs, and other expensive, hands-off diagnostic technologies, many doctors no longer feel confident doing hands-on physical exams. As a result, this change has unfortunately resulted in even more misdiagnosis and overdiagnosis of FM.

Medical Mismanagement of FM

A major reason chronic pain and fatigue are frequently mismanaged by medical practitioners is that you can't treat fibromyalgia, which is a centrally mediated pain disorder, the same way you treat localized or regional pain.[11] *Centrally mediated* means that the pain originates from a dysfunction in the central nervous system, which is made up of the brain and spinal cord. In other words, fibromyalgia is a disorder involving the way the nervous system *processes* pain. Consider this: If you are on a train that stops working because of a central computer failure affecting the whole system, it won't make any difference how much the conductor on your train fiddles around with the controls. In the same way, I have seen so many patients who—in an attempt to deal with their pain— adjust the local controls while ignoring the system-wide problem.

Inevitably, this approach backfires, and it's vital to understand why. Let's say that you have what I call classic fibromyalgia (more about what that means in Chapter 3). A glitch in your central nervous system causes your body to process pain in an oversensitized way and misinterpret the signals it receives. You can't calm a misperception arising from the central nervous system by dulling it in a local region of your body, such as the muscles of your pelvis or shoulder. But that's not all. If you *are* prescribed a narcotic pain medication, it could actually worsen the problem. Why? Because over time narcotic pain medications can, paradoxically, sharply increase the *perception* of pain while also promoting dependency. Obviously, this is counterproductive. We don't want to increase the sensation of pain or, worse, cause addiction! What's more, such medications may even cause generalized pain where previously you were only hurting in one area or region. And your muscle pains may worsen when you go off these drugs or when the drugs wear off.

I am hardly alone in noticing that medications are being used inappropriately. In a review of the research literature in early 2015, the American Society of Anesthesiologists found that, despite the variety of physicians who specialize in treating pain, people "suffer unnecessarily . . . and treat their pain with medications that may be ineffective and possibly harmful."[12] No wonder so many pain sufferers wind up traveling from clinician to clinician.

In addition to the inappropriate use of painkillers, early approaches to fibromyalgia using anti-inflammatory medications failed because classic fibromyalgia, a pain processing disorder, is not caused by substantial systemic inflammation. Then doctors tried muscle relaxants, which didn't work either because fibromyalgia is not caused by muscle tension (it's a *perception* of pain in the muscles). What tended to work the best were antidepressants—and this was discovered almost by accident: Since many patients had sleep disturbances, it was found that the tricyclic antidepressants (named tricyclic after their chemical structure, which contains three rings of atoms) used to help with their sleep also sometimes helped with their pain.

Currently, three medications, all aimed at the central nervous system, have been approved by the FDA for treating fibromyalgia.[13]

Savella (milnacipran HCl) is a serotonin and norepinephrine reuptake inhibitor (SNRI), similar to some drugs that are used to treat depression and other psychiatric disorders. Many patients who actually have classic FM, a central pain-processing disorder, experience a short-term benefit from this medication. However, it won't help those with the ailments commonly misdiagnosed as FM.

Let's look at the common side effects of Savella. These include nausea, vomiting, upset stomach, bloating, dry mouth, constipation, loss of appetite, dizziness, drowsiness, tired feeling, increased sweating, headache, hot flashes (flushing), swelling in the hands or feet, sleep problems (insomnia), weight changes, decreased sex drive, impotence, or difficulty having an orgasm.

That's not all. When compared to placebos, antidepressants increase the risk of suicidal thinking and behavior in children, adolescents, and young adults. And these drugs can be associated with other psychiatric conditions and unusual behavior and mood changes—including new or worsening anxiety, panic attacks, trouble sleeping, irritability, hostile/angry feelings, impulsive actions, severe restlessness, and very rapid speech. Wouldn't it be far better to avoid these drugs when it's possible to do so?

Duloxetine hydrochloride (Cymbalta) is also a serotonin and norepinephrine reuptake inhibitor, an antidepressant prescribed for anxiety disorder and neuropathic pain. The FDA requires that Cymbalta carry a black-box warning about the increased risk of suicide among people who use it, especially for those 24 years old or younger. Nausea, somnolence, dizziness, and insomnia are reported in 10 to 20 percent of patients. Just as with Savella, patients who actually have classic FM may benefit, at least in the short term, from this medication. However, those misdiagnosed as having FM won't experience relief and may suffer unnecessarily from this medication's possible side effects.

Pregabalin (Lyrica) is an alpha-2-delta ligand antiepileptic drug, also called an anticonvulsant. It's a gamma-aminobutyric acid (GABA) analogue, meaning it resembles this neurotransmitter and can dock in its receptors in the nervous system. (In Chapter 4, page 103, I will reveal how natural forms of GABA can help classic FM and anxiety disorders.) Lyrica works by slowing down impulses in the brain that cause seizures. It also affects chemicals in the brain that send pain signals across the nervous system. The two most common side effects are dizziness and sleepiness. Other common side effects include dry mouth, swelling of the hands and feet, blurred vision, weight gain, trouble concentrating, and feeling high.

These antidepressant and antiseizure medications can sometimes make people feel like zombies. Patients who are unnecessarily prescribed these drugs report that they are "not themselves" and may feel "numbed out," confused, or even suicidal. One of my patients said, "I find myself just driving right by my exit instead of getting off the highway even though I have lived in the same place for fifteen years." Since this frightened her, she came to me seeking ways to get off this medication and return to her normal self.

However, it should be noted that, just as with the other approved medications, Lyrica can benefit some people who actually do have classic FM. As part of a comprehensive treatment for those with a central pain-processing disorder, I sometimes suggest a trial of one of these medications. This is a different approach than that of a doctor who "reflexively" prescribes a medication because he is uninformed or does not take the time to adequately diagnose the patient.

For further discussion of medications used to treat fibromyalgia, see Chapter 4 (page 84).

Diagnosing Fibromyalgia

Far too often, busy physicians overlook one basic diagnostic principle: For a patient to be diagnosed with fibromyalgia, there can be no other explanation for their pain. And that's the tricky part. Technically, a patient could meet *all* of the 2010 ACR guidelines (page 80) even though there's a better explanation than FM for her pain. That is why it's vital to get a comprehensive overview of the person's health. Sadly, I have seen many people who were diagnosed by their primary care doctors (and even by rheumatologists and other medical specialists), who got it wrong because they missed the big picture and failed to rule out other possibilities.

There is no single objective medical test that says, "You have fibromyalgia." Therefore, doctors should make this diagnosis only after conducting a comprehensive medical history (and examination) and ruling out all other possible causes. When looking at a patient's illness, sometimes the doctor must find out what it's *not*—along with what it is. This is what doctors call a diagnosis by exclusion. And in this book, you'll be following these same exclusionary principles by answering various questions about your specific symptoms and experiences.

To eliminate the possibility of illnesses that can mimic the pain and fatigue of fibromyalgia—including hypothyroidism, autoimmune disease, anemia, mitochondrial energy insufficiency, musculoskeletal disorders, and others—I always take a thorough patient history, perform a comprehensive physical exam, and often order both standard and functional laboratory testing before making a diagnosis.

It's also important to assess how widespread the pain actually is. If the pain is regional (even if it is in multiple areas of the body), it's not fibromyalgia. The pain must be global, which means pain or achy sensations over the entire body. I also like to know how much it's affecting that person's life.

To get started, in a notebook or file on your computer, write down today's date and the answers to these questions. (You can also download a copy of them at FibroFix.com.) Answer the same questions again at one-week intervals as you read through this book in order to gauge your progress during your recovery.

- How widespread or global is the pain?

- How much does it affect your daily activities?

- Do you experience sleep disturbances such as insomnia or unrefreshing sleep?

- Do you have brain fog? That is, do you have difficulty thinking clearly and staying focused? Is your memory impaired?

- Do you suffer from anxiety or depression?

- Do you have or suspect you have irritable bowel syndrome?

Throughout the book, we will take a close look at these and other symptoms to help you identify contributors to fibromyalgia as well as to help you distinguish fibromyalgia-like symptoms from other stand-alone illnesses.

We will also look into any history of trauma, either physical or emotional, because trauma, especially during the formative times of the nervous system in youth, is a common trigger for the onset of classic fibromyalgia later in life. Later in the book (page 88), I offer a questionnaire that will help you get a handle on your personal history of trauma.

Although doctors rarely conduct comprehensive physical exams anymore, given my background in physical medicine, again, I feel that a good hands-on assessment really helps with an accurate diagnosis. Unfortunately, nowadays, many medical students simply assemble data and have not learned how to do a competent and thorough hands-on exam. A physical exam, for example, can determine that the pain is centrally mediated—a key requirement for diagnosing fibromyalgia. When pain derives from the central nervous system, you experience pain from stimuli that should *not* hurt. Another important hallmark of classic fibromyalgia is that you experience the pain in the soft tissues, not in the joints. And you hurt whenever the physician squeezes or puts digital pressure on your soft tissues, and not just in certain areas or regions.

Tender Points

There is another important distinction that can only be made with a physical exam: locating the so-called tender points of fibromyalgia, points that are perceived as painful even though there's no actual damage to (or inflammation of) the underlying local tissue. Tender points have often been used to diagnose fibromyalgia. The original 1990 American College of Rheumatology diagnostic criteria held that a person had to exhibit tenderness in at least 11 of the prescribed 18 points tested in order to receive this diagnosis. While this has since been revised to eliminate the tender point examination, tender points remain a key way to confirm global pain as opposed to local pain in one or more areas. Tender points are localized areas of tenderness in the muscles, often *around* joints but not in the joints themselves. And, as I've said, there's no apparent cause for the pain—no inflammation or injury and no knot or tightness in the muscle tissue that can be felt by the doctor. When someone presses these points with a finger, you'll flinch or pull back. They are perceived as deep areas of pain or else seem to be just under the surface of the skin. And the actual area of maximum tenderness is small, about the size of a penny.

Why did the ACR originally stipulate that there must be 11 out of 18 points for a diagnosis of fibromyalgia? Why not 12? What separated someone with 10 from 11? And how did the ACR arrive at these guidelines? I once read the meeting transcripts to learn why, and I was amazed to discover that, in fact, a bunch of rheumatologists sitting in a conference room debated back and forth and eventually compromised on the number. One doctor said 15, another said 20, and they literally *negotiated* the diagnosis. So let's just say the tender-point guidelines are a little fuzzy around the edges.

In addition, if you put pressure on many common pain points, as shown in Figure 1.2, most people will experience pain due to muscle stress, spasm, and *trigger* points (discussed in the next section below). Pain can also arise from poor posture and other daily stresses and activities such as sitting at a computer, typing on a keyboard, driving, and performing repetitive motions during work and exercise. So, yes, finding out if someone has pain or tender areas all over the body is important, but counting the exact number of tender points generally is not.

FIGURE 1.2 TYPICAL TENDER-POINT EXAMINATION SHEET

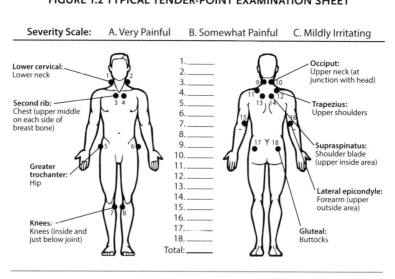

Tender Points versus Trigger Points

Tender points are not to be confused with what are known as trigger points, which are linked to an entirely different musculoskeletal condition known as myofascial pain syndrome, which has nothing to do with fibromyalgia.[14] Trigger points entail anatomical changes to muscle tissue, along with possible spasms and adhesions of the fascia, the soft tissue covering your muscles. When your fasciae are stressed from overuse or trauma, they tear and adhere to each other, preventing your muscles from working properly. Trigger points typically lead to stiff and painful muscles and decreased range of motion.

In addition, discomfort from trigger points can radiate out from the main site of the knot in the muscle. Doctors often call this "referred pain" because it comes from a chronically injured area. For example, a compressed spinal disc and a large joint, such as the shoulder, each generate distinct types of referred pain. When several kinds of referred pain overlap, these regional pain patterns can be misinterpreted as "widespread"—one of the criteria for a fibromyalgia diagnosis.[15]

It must be stressed again that trigger points also *feel* different to the touch than tender points. Trigger points have a distinct texture and feel like knots or nodules under a tight band of muscle tissue. Tender points, on the other hand, do not have any distinct textural abnormalities; they simply feel tender to the person.

Despite the fundamental differences between the two, many doctors are themselves confused and spread misinformation about this key distinction. I have seen medical textbooks as well as papers in peer-reviewed medical journals confuse the two. This signals to me that one can't trust any other information presented there. If the author can't get this basic distinction right, how will he or she understand the other more complicated nuances? I have also seen a device advertised in a major magazine for FM patients that claims to treat "the trigger points activated by fibromyalgia." And many physicians' Web sites proudly proclaim that they have great success in treating these same trigger points of FM. Again, tender points are key to diagnosing fibromyalgia—trigger points are not. *Fibromyalgia is not a muscle disorder with trigger points; it's a global pain syndrome with tender points.*

Other Misinformation

I've seen claims on doctors' Web sites that fibromyalgia is caused by hypothyroidism. Indeed, many patients who have undiagnosed hypothyroidism have been told that they have fibromyalgia. But that does not mean that fibromyalgia is *caused* by hypothyroidism. I have even seen more outrageous claims, like the assertion that fibromyalgia is caused by bacterial biofilms, a group of cells that stick together to form a coating, even though there's no evidence for this. And I have also seen claims that fibromyalgia is an autoimmune inflammatory disorder, which is

MEDICAL SYMPTOMS QUESTIONNAIRE

Name _____ Date _____

Rate each of the following symptoms based upon your typical health profile for:

☐ Past 30 days ☐ Past 48 hours

Point Scale

0 - Never or almost never have the symptom

1 - Occasionally have it, effect is not severe

2 - Occasionally have it, effect is severe

3 - Frequently have it, effect is not severe

4 - Frequently have it, effect is severe

HEAD

_____ Headaches

_____ Faintness

_____ Dizziness

_____ Insomnia   Total _____

EYES

_____ Watery or itchy eyes

_____ Swollen, reddened or sticky eyelids

_____ Bags or dark circles under eyes

_____ Blurred or tunnel vision (does not include
near or far-sightedness)   Total _____

EARS

_____ Itchy ears

_____ Earaches, ear infections

_____ Drainage from ear

_____ Ringing in ears, hearing loss   Total _____

NOSE

_____ Stuffy nose

_____ Sinus problems

_____ Hay fever

_____ Sneezing attacks

_____ Excessive mucus formation   Total _____

MOUTH/THROAT

_____ Chronic coughing

_____ Gagging, frequent need to clear throat

_____ Sore throat, hoarseness, loss of voice

_____ Swollen or discolored tongue, gums, lips

_____ Canker sores   Total _____

SKIN

_____ Acne

_____ Hives, rashes, dry skin

_____ Hair loss

_____ Flushing, hot flashes

_____ Excessive sweating   Total _____

HEART

_____ Irregular or skipped heartbeat

_____ Rapid or pounding heartbeat

_____ Chest pain   Total _____

LUNGS			
	_____	Chest congestion	
	_____	Asthma, bronchitis	
	_____	Shortness of breath	
	_____	Difficulty breathing	Total _____

DIGESTIVE TRACT			
	_____	Diarrhea	
	_____	Constipation	
	_____	Bloated feeling	
	_____	Belching, passing gas	
	_____	Heartburn	
	_____	Intestinal/stomach pain	Total _____

JOINTS/MUSCLE			
	_____	Pain or aches in joints	
	_____	Arthritis	
	_____	Stiffness or limitation of movement	
	_____	Pain or aches in muscles	
	_____	Feeling of weakness or tiredness	Total _____

WEIGHT			
	_____	Binge eating/drinking	
	_____	Craving certain foods	
	_____	Excessive weight	
	_____	Compulsive eating	
	_____	Water retention	
	_____	Underweight	Total _____

ENERGY/ACTIVITY			
	_____	Fatigue, sluggishness	
	_____	Apathy, lethargy	
	_____	Hyperactivity	
	_____	Restlessness	Total _____

MIND			
	_____	Poor memory	
	_____	Confusion, poor comprehension	
	_____	Poor concentration	
	_____	Poor physical coordination	
	_____	Difficulty in making decisions	
	_____	Stuttering or stammering	
	_____	Slurred speech	
	_____	Learning disabilities	Total _____

EMOTIONS			
	_____	Mood swings	
	_____	Anxiety, fear, nervousness	
	_____	Anger, irritability, aggressiveness	
	_____	Depression	Total _____

OTHER			
	_____	Frequent illness	
	_____	Frequent or urgent urination	
	_____	Genital itch or discharge	Total _____

GRAND TOTAL   **TOTAL** _____ wrong on both counts—it's neither an autoimmune nor a systemic inflammatory condition.

I can't emphasize enough that, because there's no clear-cut lab test for fibromyalgia, the diagnosis must be made through exclusions, or "rule outs." Fibromyalgia is the correct diagnosis only when the 2010 ACR criteria (as modified in 2011) are met; the patient's history includes many of the common, centrally mediated associated symptoms, such as irritable bowel syndrome; there is a history of high levels of stress and even trauma (in most cases); and most importantly, *all other causes have been ruled out*. Because so many patients are incorrectly labeled with fibromyalgia, I refer to the true and accurate diagnosis as classic fibromyalgia.

In a later chapter, I will ask you to complete the latest diagnostic criteria questionnaire to determine if you have classic fibromyalgia or possibly some other condition often incorrectly labeled as such. First, though, I would like you to fill out the Medical Symptoms Questionnaire. This is an instrument frequently used by physicians and other health-care providers trained in the functional-medicine approach to assess a person's overall health and vitality, or lack thereof. This will allow you to establish a baseline score on how your symptoms are impacting your health and well-being. And along with the questions you answered in the previous section, it will help you to compare your initial health status and the severity of your symptoms as you begin the program with what you'll experience after you've completed it—and once again after you put into action other interventions I will recommend, depending upon your specific needs.

You can also download a copy of this questionnaire at FibroFix.com and add it to the electronic file you have created or put it in your notebook.

Scoring: After completing the questionnaire by placing a number from 0 to 4 on each line corresponding to a symptom or set of symptoms, tally up the total for each section. This will give you an indication as to what system of the body, or grouping of symptoms, may be impacting you the most. Finally, tally up the grand total for the entire 2-page questionnaire. In general, people who are in excellent health and have good vitality score less than 25, those mildly impacted by chronic illness and metabolic dysfunction score between 25 and 50, those moderately impacted by chronic illness and metabolic dysfunction score between 51 and 100, and those who are significantly impacted by chronic illness and metabolic dysfunction score above 100. Please keep this initial score to compare with your score from this same questionnaire at the end of your 21-day program so you can assess your progress.

Conclusion

Now that you've learned why FM is so difficult to diagnose, why our health-care system is not set up to effectively treat it, and the correct way to diagnose this chronic pain disorder, it's time to begin my 21-day program of detox, diet, relaxation (stress reduction), and movement. In later chapters, we will look more deeply at classic fibromyalgia as well as the illnesses that masquerade as fibromyalgia, and you'll learn how to tell them apart. But meanwhile, by following this 21-day program, you'll start to feel better and more energetic no matter what your symptoms or their cause, and you'll begin to have the energy to actively engage in your own recovery.

CHAPTER 2

THE FIBRO-FIX
FOUNDATIONAL PLAN

In this chapter, I will share with you the Fibro-Fix Foundational Plan and everything you need to follow it over the next 3 weeks. Because the plan targets many major contributors to pain and discomfort, you will experience some immediate relief—no matter what type of pain syndrome you have. In just 3 weeks, the plan will reduce inflammation, eliminate food allergens and sensitivities, revive your low energy, and get you moving again.

Once your pain has diminished and you have more mobility and energy, you'll feel ready to take whatever additional steps are necessary to get back to vibrant health. Then, in Chapter 3, I will help you figure out the specific pain syndrome you are suffering from. And addressing the precise causes of your pain will ultimately bring further relief.

The Fibro-Fix Foundational Plan has three basic components—the anti-inflammatory and detoxifying Fibro-Fix Eating Plan, a toxin-lowering lifestyle, and gentle movement and relaxation. When you suffer from any form of chronic pain, the last thing you need is an overly complex, hard-to-follow program that adds to your stress. This three-step plan is simple, and the meals are tasty and satisfying.

First, we'll take a brief look at all three components so that you can start implementing the plan and feeling better right away! Then, we will investigate them in greater depth.

The Fibro-Fix Eating Plan

Every day for 21 days, you'll be consuming two special detox shakes, one meal, and a variety of snacks. When you suffer from any form of chronic pain, the last thing you need is an overly complex nutritional plan that adds to your stress. That is why I designed the Fibro-Fix Eating Plan to be easy to follow. The recipes (page 234) are simple, and the suggested meals are tasty. The supplements you'll take twice daily provide even more nutrients for supporting detox and lowering inflammation, while helping you to digest the additional protein you'll consume on the plan.

Like many of my patients, Leslie hated diets. "I've tried them all, trying to lose weight," she told me. The very word *diet* reminded her of the cycle of failure—the feeling of deprivation, followed by the rebound—when she went off the diet, ate all the foods she had denied herself, and put the weight back on again.

First let's be clear: The Fibro-Fix Eating Plan is not a program for losing weight. Its goal is to make you healthy, with less pain and more energy. And I designed this plan to assure that you'll never go hungry. Ample protein will help you always feel nourished. If you do experience hunger pangs, you can choose from a wide range of healthy snacks—like fruit, almond butter, nuts, and raw veggies—to eat between meals.

The good news for people like Leslie, who had sought but never achieved weight loss, is that even though the Fibro-Fix Eating Plan is not a weight-loss program, people often end up losing some weight during the course of the detox since they are taking in fewer calories and less sugar, decreasing their consumption of allergenic foods, and removing toxins from their fat stores while allowing the fat to be burned and used for energy.

A Toxin-Lowering Lifestyle

Why does a program for chronic pain seek to address toxins? No matter how hard you try to avoid them, toxins are everywhere, and they are increasing as major corporations try to push a wide range of novel chemicals on the public, whether they are proven to be safe or not. Many toxic chemicals abundant in the world today didn't even exist 30 years ago. They crop up in agriculture and food products. They are present in many consumer items. They are used in homes and buildings. They are released by industrial activities. And as part of its own internal biochemistry, the body also produces toxins that must be cleared. Because of certain metabolic dysfunctions, people with chronic pain and fatigue produce more of these internal toxins, while their mechanisms of elimination are often depressed. And once these toxins, no matter the source, find their way into the body, they become trapped in the organs and tissues, where—among many other kinds of symptoms—they can cause the fatigue and achiness that people who are labeled with fibromyalgia (FM) often experience. They also interfere with energy production at the cellular level. No wonder so many people feel tired!

Whatever the source, type, or cause of your specific pain syndrome, a simple, safe, and effective detoxification is built right into this plan's diet. You don't have to do anything special. And by doing all that I advise—drinking the shakes, eating the right foods, and taking the recommended supplements—detox happens so gently most people don't even notice it.

At the same time, there are some simple things you can do at home to help make detoxing easier. I'll detail specific recommendations later in this chapter.

Movement and Relaxation

The third element of the program is movement and relaxation—which I will explore fully in this chapter. Not enough exercise, as well as too much, can worsen pain syndromes. And I have seen people at both ends of the spectrum. Some people hope to restore their health through getting a lot of rest—but unless you have dealt with the causes of your condition, you can't rest and sleep your way out of chronic pain and fatigue. Other people try to exercise their way out. I've even had patients who were training for triathlons! Not surprisingly, this left them more depleted and exhausted than before.

You know the old adage, "No pain, no gain"? Forget it! It doesn't apply to you. Instead, the 21-day plan offers a right way to exercise. I will guide you in low-to-moderate-intensity exercises and simple stretches, alternating with rest and relaxation on days when you are feeling fatigued.

On my plan, you'll exercise with an emphasis on mobility and stretching, using gentle movement exercises as well as activities such as walking or yoga. It is important to avoid activities that overly tax your metabolic system, require a lot of exertion, or leave you out of breath. Instead, if you can tolerate it, jump on a rebounder (mini trampoline) for 3 to 5 minutes at a time. This shakes up your whole body and is particularly useful for draining your lymph system and moving those toxins out!

It's vital to reduce stress on a daily basis to resolve global pain and fatigue disorders as well as other conditions often misdiagnosed as FM. Later in the chapter, you will be introduced to simple daily practices such as progressive relaxation and guided imagery to help you reduce stress, tension, and anxiety and begin to retrain your body's response to everyday stressors.

Now, let's look at each of these elements in greater depth.

The Eating Plan

Many pain syndromes are the result of some form of inflammation. And while classic fibromyalgia, a problem arising from deep in the nervous system, is not overtly inflammatory, new evidence has emerged indicating that there is some accompanying inflammation within the microglia of the brain—the cells that act as part of the nervous system's immune defense. It's also common for people to be misdiagnosed with fibromyalgia when they really have other conditions that are caused, at least in part, by significant inflammation. That is why removing foods that can lead to inflammation, as you'll automatically do on this plan, is key.

Many people also have hidden allergies or sensitivities without realizing that some of the foods they eat may trigger a reaction. For example, my patient Julie was concerned about the dry red patches that often appeared (and disappeared) on her hands. "Am I eating too many eggs? Is it the butter I put on my toast? Or is it the wheat in the toast?" she wondered.

With food sensitivities, it can be hard to pinpoint the culprit. The link between cause and effect can be obscured by the delay between the consumption of an allergenic food and the resulting inflammatory reaction. Often, an elimination diet or testing is the only way to uncover a precise trigger. Rather than recommending that you immediately undergo time-consuming tests and self-help experiments, my plan banishes the three most common offenders when it comes to inflammation (and sensitivities)—dairy, soy, and gluten. On this plan, you'll simply remove them from your diet and see if you feel better. Most people do!

Even though the Fibro-Fix Eating Plan requires absolutely no fasting or colon cleansing—both of which can be very harsh on your system—additional features of the diet replicate the effects of fasting. Since the shakes are very satiating and you'll only consume clean foods and drinks that do not tax your digestive system, my eating plan delivers all the benefits of fasting without actually undertaking a fast. Not to mention that fasting is the last thing you need when you are already tired and in pain.

What Will I Eat?

Hundreds of people have told me that they find the plan delicious and doable. And you will be eating plenty of food. The diet consists of two pleasant-tasting, satisfying, high-protein, detoxifying, and nutrient-dense shakes per day; one regular meal per day consisting of fresh vegetables and a lean protein; and a number of supplements to improve digestion, reduce oxidative stress, promote toxin elimination, and relieve FM-like symptoms.[1]

The shakes meet a substantial portion of your baseline nutritional needs and support detox. Usually, people have the shakes for breakfast and dinner and eat lunch based on one of the meal suggestions on the menu plans. But you can easily switch it up; for example, if you prefer to eat dinner with your family, you can have the second shake at lunchtime and your meal in the evening. Or if you prefer to begin your day with a heartier breakfast, you can drink your shakes at lunch and dinner.

Keep in mind that this is not a forever program. You are not going to be replacing two meals a day with detox shakes for the rest of your life. In Chapter 8, I will provide a nutritional plan that you *can* follow for the rest of your life.

Sometimes vegans come to my practice and object to eating animal-based foods. But many vegans actually have nutritional deficiencies that compound their health problems. The reality is that to recover from chronic pain and fatigue; bypass food sensitivities; detoxify; and rebuild your nervous, gastrointestinal, and immune systems, it's best to eat abundant levels of high-quality proteins like fish and chicken, ideally from organic or natural sources. That being said, you can still follow this protocol as a vegan. The shakes that meet your baseline nutritional needs contain a vegetable protein source suitable for vegans. I will also provide vegan options for the one regular meal and snacks you'll consume each day.

The Detox Shakes

The detox shakes contain three key ingredients: a vegetable-based protein, either organic green pea protein powder or hemp protein powder; greens, either in powdered form or as fresh veggies; and a quality source of soluble and insoluble fiber. I prefer pea or hemp protein powders because many people have sensitivities to dairy proteins like whey. Rice protein, which is also frequently used in protein powders, has a number of drawbacks. It tastes bad, has a gritty texture, and contains naturally high levels of lead.

The key ingredient in my detox program is protein. Many people aren't aware of how important protein is to the detoxification process.[2] Here is why.

Detox occurs in two phases. Phase I breaks down the toxins in your body and makes them more water soluble, which readies them for the next phase. And Phase II removes them through a process called conjugation. Conjugation simply means the toxin binds with another chemical compound that will carry it out of the body. A number of substances can act as conjugators, but the most effective are sulfur-containing amino acids, which come from protein. The more protein you have in your diet, the more amino acids you have in your system, and thus the more conjugators there are on the scene to hook up with the toxins and get them out of your body.[3]

Green and Red Foods

I also recommend that patients supplement their diets with green and red foods, like organic broccoli, Swiss chard, spinach, kale, salad greens, tomatoes, beets, raspberries, and strawberries.

During the first phase of detox, when toxins are broken down, free radicals are released. It's therefore essential that antioxidants be present in your body to eliminate those free radicals. I have built ample amounts of antioxidants into the recommended foods, shakes, and supplements you'll be taking. The phytochemicals that cause foods to be green and red are the very antioxidants you need to defend against the free radicals released into the body during detox. By building your meals around these foods, you will consume even more of them. My menu plans and recipes will show you how.

Supplements

In addition to antioxidants, I recommend that my patients supplement their diets with specific nutrients that prepare the liver for detoxification, remove free radicals, and help to conjugate toxins and prepare them for safe elimination from the body. These include:

- Proteolytic enzymes, which support efficient digestion and absorption of protein
- N-acetyl-cysteine, or NAC, an antioxidant and free-radical-scavenging agent that increases glutathione at the cellular level (cysteine is also one of the sulfur-containing amino acids used to conjugate toxins)[4]
- Glutathione, one of the body's most important and powerful antioxidants and detox agents[5]
- Amino acids, including, glycine, methionine, and taurine, to conjugate and eliminate toxins

To obtain these and other supplements, go to FibroFix.com. Many of them can also be found in health food stores or obtained from health professionals. I will provide dosages later on in this chapter.

A Typical Day

On this plan, you can begin each day with an herbal tea (such as ginger, peppermint, chamomile, or hibiscus) or a decaffeinated green tea. You may also choose to drink the Morning Brew (recipe below), which contains lemon juice, hot water, and cayenne. Wait at least 15 minutes between the hot drink and the shake (or other breakfast choice) and the recommended supplements. In the morning, you can also do some stimulating hydrotherapy by alternating hot and cold water during your shower. This helps tone up the nervous system. Water is a great natural healer, and simple and enjoyable water treatments (hydrotherapy) detoxify and nourish the nervous system. You can do some of the exercises I suggest first thing in the morning, too (or you can do them in the early

MORNING BREW

Heat some water in a kettle. Fill a cup half full of filtered water, add the juice of half a lemon and a pinch of cayenne, and stir. Fill the rest of the cup with hot water from the kettle and drink. This concoction will stimulate your liver to eliminate environmental and lifestyle toxins that would otherwise be trapped in your system for a longer time.

How this works: The vitamin C in the lemon acts as a protective antioxidant. Lemon is also known to stimulate the body's natural digestive and detoxification enzymes. Cayenne pepper stimulates the circulatory system by opening the capillaries, aiding digestion, and helping to regulate blood sugar. It stimulates your metabolism, as well, which can help you lose weight over time. And it will also help your body become just a bit more alkaline (pH imbalance has been attributed to numerous disorders as well as chronic illness).

Be sure to always buy nonirradiated varieties of all spices; irradiation negates all of the health benefits you've worked so hard to acquire.

evening or at any point in the day when you have available time).

At lunch, prepare one of the meals from the menu plan, unless you drink the shake and choose to eat your meal at suppertime. A typical meal will consist of fresh vegetables with a serving of lean animal protein, like fish, chicken, or perhaps bison. Vegans can enjoy a cooked vegetable medley and a salad with a nut dressing. Between meals, if you get hungry, you can snack on fresh vegetables (like celery, carrots, or cucumber), almond butter, or vegetable broth.

You can also include alkaline vegetable broth in your meals (see page 36). Consuming vegetable broth helps the body become a bit more alkaline. My broth contains many nourishing substances that support toxin elimination and provide protection from oxidative stress and inflammation.

At the end of the day, you can do some of the relaxation exercises I will offer later in this chapter; they are great to do as you wind down your day and prepare for sleep. Many people like to do additional hydrotherapy just prior to bedtime by soaking in a warm bath with Epsom salt, a form of magnesium. This will help the body relax, improve sleep, and provide a soothing experience for the muscles and soft tissues.

Don't forget to consume extra water while detoxifying to help flush out toxins—and expect to urinate more often than usual on this program. That's a good thing!

What You'll Need for the Diet

The easiest way to begin the plan is by visiting FibroFix.com or DrDavidBrady.com to order the Fibro-Fix Foundational Detox Box. You'll then have everything you need, other than the fresh food, to complete the program over the entire 21 days. The Fibro-Fix Foundational Detox Box includes the Fibro-Fix Detox Shake in single-serving packets, the Fibro-Fix Detox Supplement packets, and a complete step-by-step program guide.

I formulated the detoxification drink powder with a unique combination of nutrients, antioxidants, and herbs that support Phase I and Phase II of the detox process. The Fibro-Fix Detox Supplement packets support the Phase II detoxification process. These packets also contain a protein-digesting enzyme formula that helps eliminate any gastrointestinal symptoms that may arise from consuming larger amounts of protein during the detoxification program.

The Fibro-Fix Detox Supplement packets are effective not only in the conjugation and elimination of toxins but also in helping protect the liver while these toxins are mobilized for excretion. The packets are designed with specific nutrients that assist in the avoidance of toxic overload and reabsorption of harmful toxins back into the bloodstream. You'll be taking one packet of capsules twice daily along with the drink mix.

While the Fibro-Fix Foundational Detox Box is offered for your convenience, you can certainly follow this plan without using these products. Let me show you how.

At your local health food store, you can obtain the near-equivalent protein powder and supplements, but you'll have to piece things together. Vitamin shops, nutritional health-care providers, and online sellers also offer the various items. Here is what you'll need.

- Vegetable-based protein powder (for example, a pea, hemp, rice, or combination formula). This should be free of sugar, artificial sweeteners and flavors (stevia is fine as a sweetener), soy, whey/dairy, and other chemical ingredients.

- Green powder (make sure it's organic)

- Fiber powder: a nonallergenic source of soluble and insoluble fiber (that is, no gluten or grains)

- N-acetyl-cysteine capsules: generally about 750 to 1,000 milligrams per capsule

- Glutathione capsules: generally about 500 milligrams per capsule

- Proteolytic enzymes capsules (protease enzymes that help support efficient digestion of protein)

- Antioxidant blend capsules: a quality blend of both water- and fat-soluble antioxidant vitamins, minerals, and herbs

As you follow the 21-day Fibro-Fix Foundational Plan, suspend any other supplements you are taking (but please check with your health-care practitioner first if he/she has recommended specific supplements).

ALKALINE BROTH: A GREAT WAY TO ADD VEGETABLES TO YOUR PROGRAM

Choose a combination of the following vegetables equaling approximately 1½ to 2 cups: celery, green beans, zucchini, spinach, parsley, kale, chard, carrots, onion, garlic, and your favorite spices. Place the vegetables in a soup pot with a significant amount of filtered water (more than enough to cover the veggies). Bring to a boil and then simmer for 45 minutes. Strain and keep the broth. You may drink as much of this broth as you want during the 21-day detoxification program, ideally at least 1 cup per day. This recipe will keep in the refrigerator for 3 days. Please do not freeze and defrost since the broth will lose some of its nutritional value. Make fresh as needed. You may also puree the vegetables and broth together in a blender to make a heartier soup.

You should also continue to take any prescribed medications. Ask your health-care practitioner if you have specific questions.

General Eating Guidelines

To get the full benefit of the program, focus on whole and seasonal foods. This usually means shopping the outer aisles of your grocery store or visiting your local farmers' market. And avoid processed and packaged foods whenever possible. (See Table 2.1 for specific food recommendations.) Here are some other basic guidelines to follow.

Stick with organic foods if possible. If they're not available, Table 2.1 lists the safest conventionally grown produce choices.

Limit starchy veggies, such as potatoes and corn, and choose lean, clean, quality protein, like chicken, bison, or fish. Avoid fish known to be high in mercury, including tuna and swordfish. Cold-water fish (preferably wild rather than farm-raised) are acceptable.

Make sure to drink ½ ounce per pound of body weight of purified water each and every day for the entire 21-day plan.

You will be eliminating sugars, desserts, and artificial sweeteners (toxic chemicals themselves), although natural low-impact sweeteners, such as stevia and polyols (xylitol and erythritol), are allowed. Some people, however, do not tolerate well the xylitol and erythritol and can get gas and cramping from them. In addition, you'll stay away from the following:

- All dairy products, such as milk, cheese, ice cream, and yogurt

- All alcohol and caffeine-containing beverages, including coffee, tea, soda, and energy drinks

- Gluten, found in wheat, rye, spelt, kamut, bulgur, couscous, and barley and in products made from these grains, including pastas, breads, crackers, and cereals. Instead, during the detox program, eat the following gluten-free whole grains in moderation.

BROWN RICE	QUINOA	STEEL-CUT OATS, OR OATMEAL
WILD RICE	AMARANTH	MARKED AS
MILLET	BUCKWHEAT	GLUTEN-FREE

What to Expect

By supporting the body's natural two-phase process of detoxification, as you will by following my plan, toxins can be cleansed from the body without discomfort. But while your metabolism is cleaning out, it may take a couple of days for your cravings to quiet down and your neurotransmitters to stop screaming at you to eat things you may be used to that aren't permitted on the plan. If you are accustomed to consuming a lot of caffeine and sugar, you may feel a slight withdrawal headache. To minimize discomfort, gradually decrease your intake of sugar and caffeine the week before going on the plan.

The protein powder and other recommended supplements will also assist your body in cleansing itself of these substances as quickly and efficiently as possible. But keep in mind that I have specifically designed the Fibro-Fix Foundational Plan to minimize discomfort by providing all the substances that keep the detox pathways running efficiently. In fact, I have more of a problem getting people *off* the diet after 21 days than I do getting them to go on it.

TABLE 2.1: FOOD AND DRINK RECOMMENDATIONS FOR THE 21-DAY PLAN

PRODUCE		PROTEIN	
ORGANIC OPTIONS	**SAFEST NONORGANIC OPTIONS**	**BEST PROTEIN OPTIONS**	**FISH TO AVOID**
• Bell peppers • Celery • Kale/collard greens • Low-glycemic fruits, fresh or frozen: Apples, apricots, blueberries, cherries, grapefruit, kiwifruit, mango, melons, nectarines, oranges, peaches, pears, plums, prunes, raspberries, strawberries, tangerines • Potatoes (in limited amounts) • Spinach	• Asparagus • Avocado • Cabbage • Eggplant • Grapefruit • Honeydew melon • Kiwifruit • Mango • Onions • Papaya • Pineapple • Sweet peas • Sweet potatoes • Watermelon	• Cold-water fish (choose wild over farm-raised): Butterfish, cod, Pacific flounder/sole, salmon, sardines, trout • Organic/hormone-free lean meats: Chicken, turkey, lamb, grass-fed beef • Organic eggs • Organic legumes	• Halibut • King mackerel • Shark • Swordfish • Tilefish • Tuna steak

The 21-Day Simple Schedule

BREAKFAST

1. Have an herbal tea (such as ginger, peppermint, chamomile, or hibiscus), decaffeinated green tea, or the lemon-honey-cayenne Morning Brew (page 33).

2. Eat breakfast or make the Fibro-Fix Detox Shake using the single-serving drink packet or the following:

25 to 30 grams vegetable-based protein powder

1 tablespoon green powder

1 tablespoon fiber

Mix in 8 to 10 ounces of water or your choice of unsweetened almond milk, coconut milk, rice milk, or another milk alternative. (See how to liven up your shakes on page 40.)

CONDIMENTS	OILS AND FATS	BEVERAGES
• Flaxseed oil or olive oil and raw apple cider vinegar for dressings • Fresh herbs and spices • Garlic • Ground red pepper • Lemon • Lime • Sea salt	• Avocado • Coconut oil for higher-heat cooking • Extra virgin olive oil • Flaxseed oil • Ghee • Hempseed oil • Organic cultured butter • Raw, sprouted, or dry-roasted nuts and seeds • Walnut oil	• Coconut water • Green juices • Herbal teas • Naturally decaffeinated green tea • Spring water

3. Take one Fibro-Fix Foundational Detox Supplement packet or the following:

   N-acetyl-cysteine: Approximately 1,000 milligrams

   Glutathione: Approximately 500 milligrams

   Proteolytic digestive enzymes: 2 capsules

   Antioxidant blend: 1 to 2 capsules

LUNCH

Eat a regular meal. For healthy gluten- and dairy-free meal suggestions, see the list on page 43. (You can also have one of your two shakes for lunch, as previously mentioned.)

DINNER

1. Make the Fibro-Fix Foundational Detox Shake using the single-serving drink packet or the following:

JAZZ UP YOUR DETOXIFICATION SHAKES

There are endless combinations of detox shakes to enjoy! Try mixing 1 packet of the Fibro-Fix Foundational Detox Shake powder (or your favorite protein powder) with:

- 8 to 10 ounces water or your choice of unsweetened almond milk, coconut milk, rice milk, or another milk alternative
- ½ to ¾ cup fresh or frozen fruit and/or vegetables: apples, berries (blackberries, blueberries, raspberries, strawberries), cherries, citrus (grapefruit, orange, tangerine), kiwifruit, mango, peaches, papaya, pineapple, and/or melon (cantaloupe, honeydew, or watermelon)
- 5 or 6 ice cubes (if not using frozen fruit)

Blend all together. Enjoy!

- **Need it sweeter?** Start with 1 packet of stevia or 1 teaspoon local raw organic honey. Adjust to your liking.
- **Like it thicker?** Add one of the following healthy options: ¼ of an avocado; a spoonful of raw almonds, raw cashews, or almond or cashew nut butter; or 1 tablespoon chia seeds.
- **Want to make it even healthier?** Throw in a handful of spinach leaves, kale, or a few raw baby carrots.
- **Want to add some zest or spice?** Use a squeeze of lemon or lime or a pinch of cinnamon, fresh ginger, or turmeric.

Need a Chocolate Fix? Try the following recipe.

- 8 to 10 ounces water or your choice of unsweetened almond milk, coconut milk, rice milk, or another milk alternative
- 5 or 6 ice cubes
- 1 packet of the Fibro-Fix Foundational Detox Shake powder (or your own favorite protein powder)
- 2 tablespoons raw cacao powder or organic cocoa powder
- 1 to 2 packets of stevia or raw honey to taste
- Optional: Add 1 tablespoon raw almond butter

25 to 30 grams vegetable-based protein powder

1 tablespoon green powder

1 tablespoon fiber

Mix in 8 to 10 ounces of water or your choice of unsweetened almond milk, coconut milk, rice milk, or another milk alternative. (See how to liven up your shakes on the opposite page.)

2. Take one Fibro-Fix Foundational Detox Supplement packet or the following:

N-acetyl-cysteine: Approximately 1,000 milligrams

Glutathione: Approximately 500 milligrams

Proteolytic digestive enzymes: 2 capsules

Antioxidant blend: 1 to 2 capsules

SNACKS

This is not a calorie-restrictive plan. If you get hungry between meals, snack on healthy whole foods in moderation, including nuts (preferably raw and not peanuts), hummus (unless it gives you excessive gas), raw or steamed vegetables, and low-glycemic fruit. If you need a snack, by all means eat one. Waiting too long to respond to a hunger pang can lead you to eat more than you really need. At the same time, see if a small snack (one apple instead of three) will satiate you before you eat more. To do this, you will need to tune in to your body and make sure that you are truly hungry, not just bored, tired, or stressed.

MENU IDEAS

To follow are some sample meal plans to give you a full range of choices for foods you can enjoy on the Fibro-Fix Foundational Plan. You will find options for meat eaters, vegans, and those who are gluten-free or dairy-free. While I offer some general instructions for food preparation for some of the recommended dishes, you will find complete recipes later in

LOW-GLYCEMIC FRUIT

A food's glycemic load (GL) is calculated using a measurement called the *glycemic index*, which defines how much a food raises blood sugar levels. By simply taking the food's glycemic index, dividing it by 100, and multiplying it by the grams of carbohydrates (excluding fiber) in a typical serving size, you can calculate its GL. A GL of above 20 is considered high, 11 to 19 is considered average, and below 11 is low. Fruits with a low glycemic load include:

Apples	Kiwifruit	Pineapple
Apricots	Mango	Plums
Blueberries	Nectarines	Prunes
Cantaloupe	Oranges	Strawberries
Grapefruit	Peaches	Watermelon
Guava	Pears	

this book. Remember that two meals per day should be replaced by shakes. (The recipe section contains some creative ways to vary your shakes.)

SAMPLE BREAKFAST OPTIONS

2 to 3 hard-boiled eggs with ½ grapefruit
⅔ cup hot quinoa cereal or gluten-free steel-cut oats, 1 scoop protein powder (about 8 to 10 grams), ½ cup berries, and a small handful of walnuts or pecans
Breakfast Detox Scramble: Scramble 2 to 3 eggs with onion and/or garlic and/or broccoli.
Add leftover salmon from the night before to sautéed veggies, stir to heat up, and add condiments/spices.
2 to 3 poached eggs over a bed of fresh spinach and sliced tomato
2 to 3 slices turkey bacon with leftover veggies from the night before or sliced tomato and avocado

Green salad with sprouts, extra virgin olive oil, basil, and a squeeze of lemon or lime

Baked cod topped with avocado salsa: To make the salsa, mix together 1 avocado, chopped; 1 tomato, chopped; $1/2$ cup chopped red onion; $1/2$ cup capers (drained); $1/4$ cup chopped fresh cilantro; $1/2$ teaspoon cumin; $1/8$ teaspoon ground red pepper; and 2 tablespoons lime juice.

1 cup black bean soup

Cabbage and chicken salad: Toss leftover chopped grilled chicken with shredded cabbage and raw apple cider vinegar.

Organic vegetable broth

Shrimp and vegetables: Over medium heat, sauté fresh tail-on shrimp and chopped garlic in a pan with coconut oil. Roughly chop 5 to 10 different vegetables and lightly stir-fry with freshly grated ginger, the sautéed shrimp and garlic, and $1/2$ cup cooked buckwheat noodles. Lightly drizzle with sesame oil.

Baby greens salad with extra virgin olive oil and a squeeze of lemon or lime

Grilled buffalo burger on a baked or grilled portobello mushroom

Mixed roasted vegetables: Roast a combination of cauliflower, broccoli, and/or Brussels sprouts.

Beet greens with extra virgin olive oil and a squeeze of lemon or lime

Wild salmon, steamed or grilled

Steamed beets: Steam the beets for 20 to 30 minutes, or until soft, and then peel off the skin.

Mixed greens salad with extra virgin olive oil or lemon-flavored flaxseed oil

Broiled chicken with peppers: Roughly chop green, yellow, and red bell peppers; onion; and mushrooms. Sauté lightly with extra virgin olive oil and chopped garlic. Serve with broiled chicken and wild brown rice.

Steamed veggies (cauliflower, broccoli, carrots) drizzled with olive oil and lemon juice

Baked farm-raised wild salmon topped with tomato pesto

Roasted green beans

Grilled turkey breast with sage

$1/2$ baked sweet potato

Baked sole with lemon

$1/2$ cup baked acorn or butternut squash

Steamed green and yellow beans topped with flaxseed oil

Steamed kale

Grilled chicken with garlic pesto: Add 2 cloves garlic, minced, and $1/2$ cup finely chopped fresh basil or $1/2$ teaspoon dried basil to $1/8$ cup extra virgin olive oil. Spread the garlic-basil mixture on chicken breasts and allow to marinate while preparing the rest of dinner. Grill.

1 cup hearty vegetable soup Grilled cod, sole, or flounder Steamed artichoke with lemon
3 to 4 ounces chicken salad (made with olive oil instead of mayonnaise) wrapped in a large lettuce leaf. Add grated carrots, chopped avocado, or other veggies of your choice.
Large mixed green salad with veggies of your choice and 3 to 4 ounces grilled chicken or fish, topped with extra virgin olive oil, lemon, and herbs of your choice.
Turkey Roll-Up: Chop up tomato, cucumber, and $1/4$ avocado; grate a carrot; and add to the middle of a slice of nitrate-free turkey. Roll the turkey around the ingredients. *Variation:* Add salsa or hummus.
Vegan Options: Steamed (or lightly sautéed in olive oil) vegetable medley with lemon-sesame dressing (tahini, garlic, lemon juice, parsley, and water) Wheat-free tempeh Salad with avocado and walnuts

HEALTHY SNACK OPTIONS

1 piece fruit and 10 to 12 almonds, walnuts, or pecans
Cut up carrots or bell peppers with 1 to 2 tablespoons hummus (if tolerated)
Apple slices or celery sticks with 1 tablespoon almond butter

A Toxin-Lowering Lifestyle

By cleaning up your diet and eliminating common toxins and allergens, improving your energy production and cellular vibrancy, and reducing inflammation and achiness, you'll be well on your way to feeling better and more actively engaged in your recovery as you continue to learn about the interventions that are appropriate to your situation. That is the goal of the Fibro-Fix Eating Plan and a toxin-lowering lifestyle.

Together, these are a first-step intervention that will help with your overall health, start the process of rejuvenating your metabolism, and prepare you for recovery.

Why Remove Toxins?

There is so much confusion about toxins today, and many conventional practitioners pooh-pooh the whole notion of detox. But again, that is because they are focused on dealing with health symptoms once they become severe rather than on preventing illness. In seeking to prevent illness, functional medicine looks at the causes of health imbalances. The unprecedented dissemination of toxic substances is a major contributor to these imbalances. Our bodies were never designed to handle this overload. And it's not just when you are ill that you have to pay attention to toxins. If this topic is new to you, I will help you learn why.

Unfortunately, toxins are in the food you eat, the air you breathe, the water you drink, and the medicines you take. For example, even ordinary tap water is a potential source of chemical toxicity. The Environmental Protection Agency reported that the quality of tap water throughout North America has diminished significantly in the past few decades. Tap water is commonly contaminated with a variety of toxic chemicals, heavy metals, pesticide and herbicide residues, and even medications.

That is why your body needs to rid itself of toxins all the time. This is more challenging today than it has been for previous generations, because many of the toxins we are exposed to were unknown 50 years ago.

Some toxins are a natural by-product of your body's metabolic processes—of its basic biological functioning. When toxins, whether externally or internally derived, become trapped in the body's organs and tissues, over time they can negatively impact your health, vitality, and overall wellness. Allowed to accumulate, they can undermine your metabolism and contribute to chronic illness. That is why, on my plan, you'll help your body to detoxify as well as avoid adding to its toxic burden.

Detox: A Continuous Process

Detoxification is a continuous physiologic process that your body depends on for survival. Complex cellular detoxification mechanisms are constantly at work for you all day, every day. In the face of a virtually constant barrage of toxic material, a complex structure of cells, organs, and organ systems processes natural and synthetic chemicals to keep you healthy. That is why I recommend specific ways to help keep your body's toxic burden low and your detox mechanisms working for the long haul. Here is what I suggest.

Minimize use of plastics. Heating foods in plastic containers in microwave ovens releases harmful chemicals. You should never heat food in plastic. Use glass or ceramic instead.

Engage in skin brushing. To aid in lymphatic drainage, use a dry, natural-fiber shower brush or loofah to massage your entire body before you shower or bathe. Start at the toes and gently scrub, using circular motions, toward your heart.

Try hydrotherapy. You can do your own hydrotherapy session in the shower by alternating between hot and cold water. This stimulates circulation and your immune system. You can also do a sauna/cold shower/sauna combination if you belong to a gym. This is not for the squeamish, but you'll feel great afterward.

Take Epsom salt baths. A warm bath with Epsom salt is a great way to relax and detox. You may also rub on the salt with a warm, wet washcloth in the bath or shower. This is very invigorating. It provides a great source of topical magnesium, which can soothe the muscles and soft tissues of the body.

Use filtered water. Public tap water is often contaminated. Drink and cook with only pure filtered water, and consider adding a filter to your shower.

Avoid cooking in microwave ovens. Although the convenience of microwaves is indisputable, this method of heating can disrupt chemical linkages in otherwise healthy foods and decrease their nutritional value. Heat food on a stove top or oven whenever possible, and use a cast-iron pan. Avoid Teflon and synthetic nonstick coatings. If you use a microwave, do not overheat the food, and use glass or ceramic containers instead of plastic ones.

Movement and Relaxation

The strategies in the previous section for incorporating detox into your everyday life are an essential part of the foundational plan. Just as important is the movement and relaxation component of the plan. For understandable reasons, many people with pain syndromes have some resistance to movement and exercise. In this section, I look at the importance of movement and relaxation to both the short- and long-term healing of those who suffer from chronic pain and fatigue, and I show you ways to engage in them easily, safely, and comfortably through both movement and relaxation.

How Much Is Too Much?

Advertisements for athletic equipment or sports drinks proclaiming "Go hard or go home" lead us to imagine that the only form of exercise is high intensity and fast paced. Pictures of well-muscled athletes convince us that it isn't worth exercising if we don't get our heart rate elevated or if we aren't breathing hard and dripping with sweat when we're done.

It's true that intense activity can benefit health, but this type of activity also stresses the body. And in the short term, it causes damage and inflammation at the cellular level. That is why it's suitable for healthy, robust, well-nourished, and well-rested individuals, and even they must be careful not to overdo it. The truth is, too much exercise, too frequently, with insufficient rest and recovery and inadequate nutrition, can be just as harmful as no exercise at all. On the other hand, many people with chronic pain syndromes avoid exercise of any kind due to pain, fatigue, and reduced range of motion.

Maybe it's been months—or years—since you've even *imagined* going for a brisk walk. Some days, it might be a struggle just to make your way around your house and perform everyday chores. The pain, discomfort, and low energy associated with your FM may actually be your body's way of telling you that it is already experiencing enough strain. You may doubt you are capable of even slow, gentle movements. The mere mention of the word *exercise* may fill you with dread. If any of this is true for you, I hope this chapter will help you change your perspective on this crucial aspect of your healing.

The plan I offer will help you discover ways to move more easily than you ever thought possible. As your body clears away toxins that may be causing or exacerbating your symptoms, and as you remove foods from your diet that may be causing an unrecognized, low-level, chronic sensitivity response, the inflammation in your body will begin to subside, and you may find your body *wanting* to move more.

Your new dietary strategy will also replenish nutrient stores that may have been depleted through emotional and physiological stress, overexercising, or a diet that was not right for you. As all these factors are brought into alignment, you'll find gentle movement to be quite pleasant and restorative.

Getting Back to Movement and Relaxation

On this plan, you'll learn the following basic approaches.

- Gentle stretching and mobility exercises

- Progressive muscle relaxation

- Guided imagery for stress reduction

Only the first involves even mild exercise. The other two "exercise" the subtle connection between mind and body. You won't be sprinting up hills or getting out of breath. Rather, you'll be retraining your nervous system, allowing it to moderate its interpretation of everyday stimuli, such as lights, sounds, odors, and touch.

Mild exercise will improve bloodflow and muscle relaxation, while stress management techniques and cognitive behavioral therapies, such as meditation, yoga, and guided imagery, can help moderate your nervous system's response to everyday stimuli, helping to calm your perception of pain and reduce other symptoms.

You might be thinking, "*Great!* This makes a lot of sense. I'm on board! But how *do I do it?!*" The sections that follow will walk you through the details of each of the three strategies.

Gentle Stretching and Mobility Exercises

My friend and colleague Edward G. McKiernan, DPT, has been practicing physical therapy for over 20 years, specializing in the treatment of joint and muscle pain. I have combined my experience in physical medicine with his extensive experience to provide you with these easy-to-follow mobilization and strengthening exercises, targeting those areas responsible for bearing weight, including the neck (cervical spine), mid-back (thoracic spine), lower back (lumbar spine), hips, and knees. Along with the responsibility of bearing weight, these areas, particularly the neck and lower back, must adapt to specific work environments and activities—for example, sitting hunched over while performing computer-related tasks. This scenario can create chronic pain and lack of mobility.

Along with physical stress resulting from weight-bearing and postural changes, emotional stress can induce muscle spasms in these areas, resulting in pain, lack of mobility, fatigue, and weakness. When these muscles are in a weakened state, they can no longer support the spine and are unable to provide for a natural, healthy posture. This can lead, over time, to degenerative joint problems, which doctors call osteoarthritis.

The gentle stretching exercises presented here target pain, stiffness, and restricted range of motion. You can always increase (or decrease) the number of repetitions called for according to your own tolerance and comfort level. Also, while doing these exercises, please pay attention to your breathing. I recommend that you use diaphragmatic breathing, which I'll explain below.

For these exercises, you'll need an exercise ball, a floor mat, and a towel.

DIAPHRAGMATIC BREATHING

Instructions: Breathe through your nose and allow your stomach to expand, as opposed to your chest. Then, exhale through your mouth and allow your stomach to deflate.

(Practice by placing your hand on your stomach and feeling it inflate and deflate when taking a breath.)

1. HORIZONTAL SHOULDER STRETCH

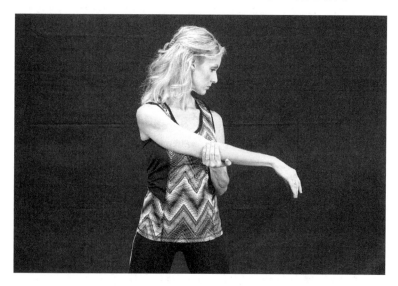

Targets: Neck, upper back, shoulders

Purpose: Increase neck, shoulder, and upper-back mobility; reduce muscle tightness; and restore normal, healthy posture

Instructions: In a standing position, with your feet shoulder-width apart and knees slightly bent, clasp your right elbow with your left hand. Bring your right arm horizontally across your body toward your left side while rotating your chin over your left shoulder. Slightly pull your right elbow with your left hand to increase your upper-back rotation to the left side just a little bit. Hold for three slow diaphragmatic breaths. This is 1 repetition. Complete 10 repetitions. Repeat the same sequence, bringing the left arm horizontally across the body and rotating the chin over the right shoulder.

2. SEATED CHIN TUCK-IN

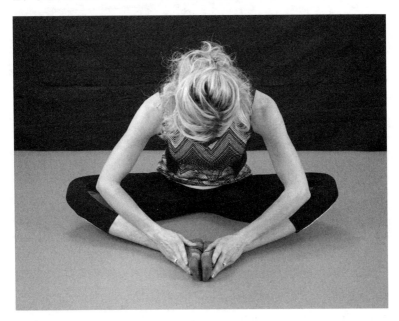

Targets: Neck, upper back, left and right groin

Purpose: Increase neck, upper-back, and groin mobility; reduce muscle tightness; and restore normal, healthy posture

Instructions: In a sitting position, with the soles of your feet pressed together and your elbows resting on your knees, tuck your chin down into your chest while bending your head forward until you feel a slight pulling sensation in your neck and upper back. While your elbows are on your knees, push your elbows down gently until you feel a slight pulling sensation in the groin area. Hold this position for three slow diaphragmatic breaths. This is 1 repetition. Repeat until you complete a total of 10 repetitions.

3. MID-BACK EXTENSION ON A BALL

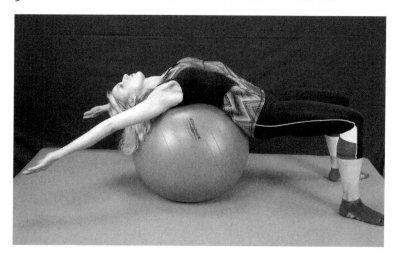

Targets: Chest, upper back, mid-back

Purpose: Increase upper-body and mid-back mobility; reduce muscle tightness; and restore normal, healthy posture

Instructions: With the exercise ball under your mid-back and both arms crossed and resting on your chest, extend both arms by reaching over your head, slightly rolling upward on the ball. Extend your legs outward. Hold this position for three diaphragmatic breaths. Return your arms to your chest. This is 1 repetition. Repeat this exercise for a total of 10 repetitions.

4. UPPER-BODY PRESS-UP

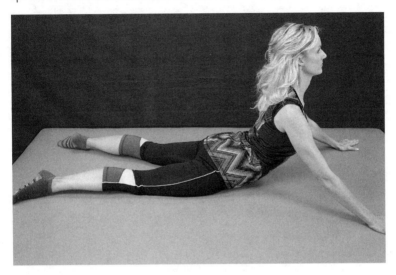

Targets: Neck, chest, upper back, lower back, pelvis

Purpose: Increase neck, upper-back, and lower-back mobility; reduce muscle tightness; and restore normal, healthy posture

Instructions: Lying on your stomach, with arms shoulder-width apart by your sides, gently press your upper body upward, extending your neck and head (looking upward), while gently pressing your pelvis downward. Stop when you feel a minimal pull (stretching sensation) in your middle and lower back. Hold this position for three diaphragmatic breaths. Return to the starting position. This is 1 repetition. Repeat this exercise for a total of 10 repetitions.

5. DOUBLE KNEE TOWARD CHEST

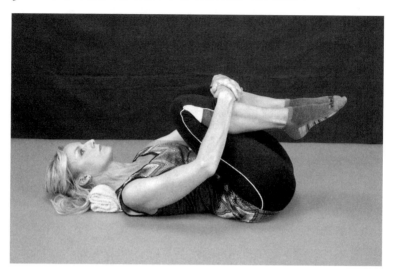

Targets: Lower back

Purpose: Increase lower-back mobility; reduce muscle tightness; and restore normal, healthy posture

Instructions: With a rolled towel placed behind your neck, lying on your back with your knees bent, bring both your knees up toward your chest by clasping them with your hands. Pull your knees toward your chest until you feel a minimal stretching sensation in your lower back. Hold this position for three diaphragmatic breaths. Return to the starting position. This is 1 repetition. Repeat for a total of 10 repetitions.

6. UPPER-THIGH STRETCH

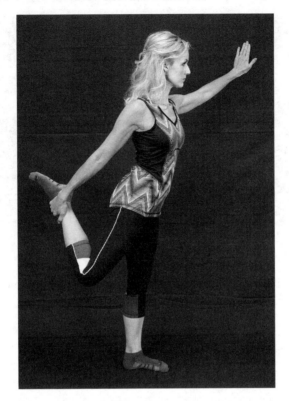

Targets: Hips, knees, ankles

Purpose: Increase hip, knee, and ankle mobility; reduce muscle tightness; and restore healthy, normal posture

Instructions: Standing next to a wall, stretch your left arm above your head, placing it on the wall, and bend your right knee, clasping your right foot with your right hand. Pull your right foot back and upward toward your buttocks until you feel a minimal stretch in your thigh. Hold this position for three slow diaphragmatic breaths, and then lower your leg to the floor. This is 1 repetition. Repeat this exercise for a total of 10 repetitions. Then repeat the same sequence with your left leg.

7. HIP EXTENSION WITH A BALL

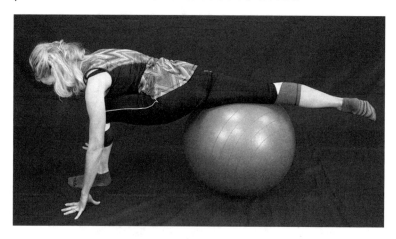

Targets: Pelvis, hips

Purpose: Increase pelvis and hip mobility; reduce muscle tightness; and restore normal, healthy posture

Instructions: With the exercise ball under your right thigh, place your left leg forward with your knee bent. Place your hands on your left knee, or if you can, flat on the floor. You should feel a minimal stretching sensation in your right upper-thigh and hip region. Hold this position for 15 seconds while engaged in diaphragmatic breathing. Increase or decrease the stretching time based on your tolerance level. Repeat this sequence once with the ball placed under your left thigh.

8. INNER-THIGH STRETCH

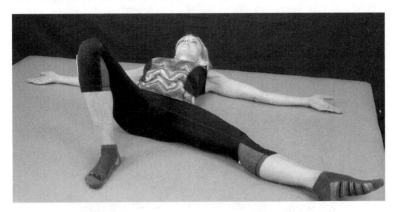

Targets: Pelvis, hips

Purpose: Increase pelvis and hip mobility; reduce muscle tightness; and restore normal, healthy posture

Instructions: Lying on your back with your arms spread out horizontally and palms facing upward, bend your right knee and keep your left leg straight. Then slide your left leg outward until you feel a minimal stretching sensation in your left inner-thigh and groin region. Hold this position for 2 minutes while breathing diaphragmatically. Increase or decrease the stretching time based on your tolerance level. Repeat the sequence once with your right leg.

9. STANDING CALF STRETCH

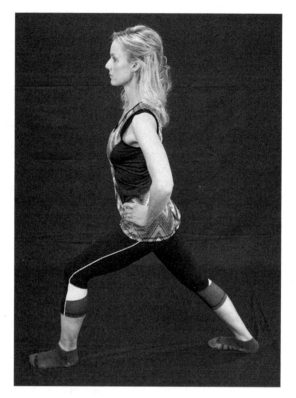

Targets: Ankles, knees

Purpose: Increase ankle and knee mobility; reduce muscle tightness; and restore normal, healthy posture

Instructions: With your hands on your hips, place your left foot in front of your right foot with your legs spread apart. Bend your left knee forward until you feel a slight stretching sensation in the right calf region. Hold this position for 1 minute while engaged in diaphragmatic breathing. Repeat the sequence by placing your right foot in front of your left and bending the right knee forward.

Why You Need to Retrain Your Nervous System

One key symptom of classic fibromyalgia is feeling bombarded by sensory input that other people barely register. Due to an overactive fight-or-flight response, your body is perpetually hypervigilant and poised for an emergency—and you might not even realize it. The goal of resetting your nervous system's response is to make outside stimuli—some of which may seem irritating or painful—easier to tolerate.

Here I will show you how to dial down your body's fight-or-flight reaction and engage its rest-and-repair response instead.

However, just as with physical exercise—say, biking or swimming—you have to work at these relaxation techniques. You have to do them regularly and make them habits. It'll take some time to learn the basics, and you may feel a little lost at first, wondering whether you're doing them well enough to reap the benefits. Remember, though, there's no right or wrong way to do them, and these gentle approaches are as crucial to your healing as anything you'll do for your physical body.

Progressive Muscle Relaxation

Progressive muscle relaxation is crucial for those living with FM and chronic pain. You might not realize how tense your body is until you engage in deliberate efforts to relax it. Muscle tension you're not aware of could be worsening your pain and stiffness. Fortunately, the mind-body connection works both ways: from the body to the mind, and from the mind to the body, enabling us to use the mind to relax the body.

A simple example of a transmission from body to mind and back to the body is when you accidentally touch a hot pan on the stove. The nerves in your hand feel the temperature and report this to the brain, and your brain tells the motor neurons in your arm muscles to pull your hand away. Of course, this all takes place in an instant; there's almost no time lag between when you first touch the dangerously hot pan and then flinch away.

But muscle tension doesn't always require an external stimulus, like that hot pan. You might be holding your muscles more tightly than necessary for no identifiable reason other than that's simply how you've always held your body. Whether seated, standing, lying down, or in motion, you might be tightening muscles that are unrelated to the movement at hand, adding extra tension where none is required. And just as the body responds to negative thoughts, worry, and anxiety by becoming tense and tight, tense and tight muscles send feedback to the brain, which can result in increased feelings of emotional stress, anxiety, and unease.

A dedicated program of progressive muscle relaxation can be helpful in both the short and the long term—that is, while you're actively doing it, and even when you're not. While you are engaging in muscle relaxation, you'll obviously be deliberately releasing tension. But in time, you'll grow accustomed to how it feels to be relaxed. Then, throughout the rest of your day, you'll be able to recognize when you are inordinately tense and make immediate corrections that will have beneficial effects on your overall well-being. The more you can train your body to be relaxed, regardless of your immediate surroundings (a traffic jam, a hectic meeting at work), the more manageable your pain and fatigue will become.

The technique is simple and is commonly performed while lying down, but you can do it seated if you prefer. In time, when you're familiar with the process, you'll be able to do it anywhere—at your desk; as a passenger in a car, train, or plane; or even while on the phone.

Until you are comfortable with the technique, try to do it in a quiet room. (Some people find progressive relaxation is easiest to do in bed before going to sleep.) Minimize distractions, such as TV, computers, and loud noises. Keep your phone in another room or turn it off so you're not distracted by incoming calls or messages. Wear comfortable clothing, and avoid performing this technique after a large meal.

It's up to you whether you prefer to proceed from your head downward or from your toes upward. The exercise is equally effective in either direction. When you're ready to begin, focus on slowing down your breathing. Then, going through each of the following areas, one by one, tense the muscles for 5 seconds, release the tension, and relax for 10 seconds.

- Feet and toes*
- Calves*
- Thighs*
- Stomach
- Back

- Shoulders*
- Arms*
- Hands*
- Neck
- Head and face

Progressive muscle relaxation will teach you to feel and understand the difference between tension and relaxation. This will help you identify tension even while not engaged in this exercise. Once you recognize what tension feels like, and you become more aware of it throughout the day, you'll be able to make immediate corrections to lessen the burden of stress on your body and mind.

Guided Imagery for Stress Reduction

Living with a chronic pain syndrome can lead you to feel gloomy about your condition and the limitations it places on your life or the lives of those close to you. Have you noticed that the more you focus on your discomfort, the more pain and unease you experience? If so, this is tangible evidence of the mind-body connection at work.

Breaking out of this vicious cycle isn't as simple as just putting on a happy face or "faking it 'til you make it." Establishing new, helpful thought patterns requires time and dedication, but its benefits can be as profound as those of a healthy diet, targeted supplementation, or any medication.

Guided imagery is a powerful tool to help you reconnect with optimism, positive thoughts, and all the ways in which your body *is* working well. According to the prestigious Cleveland Clinic, "guided imagery is a form of focused relaxation that helps create harmony between the mind and body. It's a way of focusing your imagination to create calm, peaceful images in your mind, thereby providing a 'mental escape.'"[6] Research has shown that guided imagery can reduce depression, pain, stress, and anxiety as well as deepen your sleep,

---

* For these muscle groups, you can tighten and loosen your left and right sides at the same time, but you might find yourself more attuned to your body by doing them separately.

increase relaxation, and enhance healing and quality of life.

You can harness the power of guided imagery anytime, anywhere, even in the midst of acute stress. In fact, you have probably engaged in guided imagery all of your life—for example, salivating as you imagine your favorite food or getting excited thinking about someone you're sexually attracted to. These are instances of your *psychology* influencing your *physiology*.

Next, I will offer several guided imagery scenarios that you can customize to appeal to you. The key is to find images and scenarios that *you* enjoy and that are relaxing for *you*. There is no dogma or "right" or "wrong" way to engage in guided imagery. It's simply a strategy to help you tune into the part of your mind that holds inner calm and joy, where you are energetic, vibrant, and well.

Breathing in Peace. Imagine a relaxing, peaceful setting, and with this image in your mind, focus on your breathing, keeping it deep, calm, and unhurried.

Slow and Soften. Focus on slowing your heart rate and reducing musculoskeletal tension, as if your bones have turned to Jell-O and all of your tender points have softened.

Five Senses Centering. Picture yourself in a calm and beautiful place. Now, in your imagination, try to incorporate input to all five senses. See the place, hear its natural sounds, feel the breeze on your skin, smell the nearby plants or flowers, taste the water in that nearby brook. Integrating the sensory input makes the experience more tactile and may help you more deeply engage in it and relax.

Bubble Bath Sensations. Imagine yourself in a bubble bath. Feel the warm, soapy water dissolving the tension in your body. Smell the fragrance and visualize the soft, amber glow of the candles you've lit in the room. Maybe there's some soft classical music playing, and you can hear that while you taste the wine or dark chocolate you're treating yourself to.

Sweet Sounds Relaxation. You might find that you can access your "inner sanctum" more easily in the presence of calming sounds. Pick ones that appeal to you, such as a gently rolling stream, a summer rain, song birds in a forest, or calming Native American flutes.

Remember, when it comes to guided imagery, there are no hard-and-fast rules. The only requirement is finding something that works for *you* and doing it consistently for about 10 minutes every day. The point is to relax and de-stress. If you find yourself feeling *more* agitated because you think you're "doing it wrong," please try to remove feelings of self-judgment. You are in a process of healing. *Be kind to yourself.* Guided imagery and relaxation exercises can be done for 20 to 30 minutes a day.

If you would like some initial education on how to start a practice of guided meditation, there are numerous helpful CDs or online audio downloads. Audio programs available at healthjourneys.com provide the imagery so that you can just listen and relax. You can also seek out a guided imagery practitioner in your area to help you create your own routine.

Above all, be patient with yourself. It may take some time before you are able to identify tense versus relaxed muscles or to walk yourself through a pleasant scenario in your mind. The important thing is to do these exercises in a way that works for you—or consider seeking alternative stress reduction and relaxation methods, such as meditation, tai chi, or yoga.

New patterns of physical movement—walking, riding a bicycle, dancing—become second-nature after an initial period of learning and practicing. So will the new patterns and responses you cultivate through this plan. Even in the midst of a stressful situation, you'll be able to preserve peace and calm in your body and mind.

For more ideas on techniques for relaxation and stress reduction, see FibroFix.com.

Conclusion

In this chapter, you learned about and began to follow the three elements of the Fibro-Fix Foundational Plan—the anti-inflammatory and detoxifying Fibro-Fix Eating Plan, a toxin-lowering lifestyle, and gentle movement and relaxation—that will allow you to feel better immediately, no matter what the cause of your symptoms.

In the next chapter, you will learn how to tell the difference between classic fibromyalgia and the illnesses that are all too often mistaken for it, and you will answer questions about your specific symptoms and history. You are finally on your way to understanding, and dealing with, the true source of your chronic pain and fatigue.

CHAPTER 3

DO YOU HAVE FIBROMYALGIA— OR SOMETHING ELSE?

People who come to my clinic often ask me how their doctors missed what was going on with them. It's not that surprising when you realize fibromyalgia has only recently been recognized as a bona fide health condition. And most health-care providers are still very unclear about this ailment and its mimics. That's why all too many people encounter confusion, and unfortunately often dismissal and ridicule, when they seek help for their chronic pain syndrome.

- Diagnosed with fibromyalgia, Judy suffered from widespread pain and fatigue and was unable to lose weight. After 2 years of unsuccessfully trying different pain and antidepressant medications, she finally got a second opinion and was diagnosed with a thyroid gland problem. After she started taking thyroid medication, her so-called fibromyalgia pain went away completely.

- Jeff suffered from terrible fatigue and achiness throughout his body, especially in his legs. A doctor diagnosed him with fibromyalgia and gave him an antidepressant. Over the years, I have seen several people with the leg weakness that Jeff suffered from. In some instances, they were taking cholesterol-lowering drugs known as statins. A common side effect of these medications is muscle weakness and pain. Jeff spoke to his cardiologist, and the doctor decided to take him off Lipitor. Instead, he went on the Fibro-Fix Eating Plan and started taking fish oil, niacin, and a standardized red yeast rice supplement. Because the eating plan is anti-inflammatory and features healthy fats and eliminates simple carbohydrates, it can modulate cardiac risk factors in the majority of cases. And research shows that the supplements on the plan can support healthy cholesterol levels and reduce cardiovascular risks, as well. This type of treatment is often well tolerated even by those who seem to have side effects when taking cholesterol-lowering medications. That turned out to be the case for Jeff. Within 2 months, his "fibromyalgia" pain went away. His muscle aches and fatigue were never really fibromyalgia to begin with, just common side effects of statin medications.

- Kim experienced pain in multiple joints. When her doctor ordered tests to determine if she suffered from rheumatoid arthritis, the results came back negative. Her doctor then told her that she had fibromyalgia and put her on pain medications. After a few months, Kim went to a rheumatologist who did new blood tests and found inflammation markers. More blood tests confirmed that Kim had lupus. Kim followed a comprehensive functional medicine treatment for this autoimmune disorder. Once she had addressed the lupus, her pain went away completely.

- Betty was diagnosed with fibromyalgia after her doctor couldn't find any other explanation for her fatigue and widespread pain. She mentioned that her symptoms worsened after her husband was diagnosed with prostate cancer. Her doctor recommended that she take a muscle relaxant before bedtime to improve her sleep and a low-dose antidepressant to help reduce her anxiety. After she started the Fibro-Fix Foundational Plan and incorporated other treatments discussed later in this book, Betty's pain receded. And after she discontinued the medications, which made her feel drowsy and spacey, Betty started to feel normal again. Although medications can sometimes be helpful, in Betty's case, they provided little relief and produced undesirable side effects instead.

Although all four people had been diagnosed with fibromyalgia, it turned out that Judy, Jeff, and Kim had other medical problems that were causing their symptoms of widespread pain and fatigue. Judy had an underactive thyroid condition, Jeff was experiencing a common reaction to cholesterol-lowering medications, and Kim had an autoimmune disease. None of them had fibromyalgia. Only Betty was suffering from classic fibromyalgia. A significant clue, in her case, was the stress she was currently experiencing in her life. FM can result from a pattern of traumatic or stressful events early in life, when the nervous system is forming, and then be triggered by stressful or traumatic events in the present.

Fortunately, each of these stories had a happy ending. But that's not always the case. Many people suffer for years with the wrong diagnosis and take the wrong medications, feeling more and more helpless and defeated. Fibromyalgia can't be cured, they are told. "You should just try to manage it" is the all-too-frequent advice. Some doctors contend that fibromyalgia is not real and urge patients to simply get over it and go on with their lives.

In reality, the typical FM diagnosis is just an oversimplified scheme that lumps together many entirely different conditions simply because they happen to share a common cluster of symptoms. This is like equating a headache, an earache, and a stuffy nose—because they all take place in the head! Used too broadly, the term *fibromyalgia* fails to answer important questions, like:

- Why do some patients benefit from low-dose antidepressants while others feel worse or experience no effect from taking them?

- Why does manual therapy—such as massage, physical therapy, or chiropractic treatment—work with some patients and not others?

- Why are dietary changes, vitamins, and herbal remedies successful in relieving the achiness, gastrointestinal symptoms, and fatigue of some cases of FM but not all?

- And why are some patients but not others dramatically "cured" of their FM symptoms when placed on thyroid or other hormone-replacement therapies?

The bottom line is that only a small number of patients diagnosed with FM actually suffer from the classic variety of this syndrome.[1] Most are really suffering from another problem. In fact, according to the medical literature, there's an error rate of 66 percent or more in the diagnosis of fibromyalgia.[2]

In most cases, the source of the chronic pain and fatigue can be found in one of three common categories of health problems, or "buckets."

1. **Musculoskeletal issues.** The body's musculoskeletal system is made up of bone, muscle, fascia, cartilage, tendons, ligaments, joints, and other connective tissues. Common musculoskeletal problems that may lead to a misdiagnosis of FM include the "muscle knots" (or trigger points) found in myofascial pain syndrome; spinal joint problems, such as disc degeneration; spinal canal narrowing (stenosis); tendonitis; and pinched nerves from disc bulges; herniations; or bony overgrowths from degenerative osteoarthritis.

2. **Functional problems.** Your body is processing chemical reactions in the cells, organs, and systems all the time. This metabolic activity allows the body to maintain and repair itself and to grow, reproduce, and interact. Among the most important cellular structures engaged in metabolic activity are the mitochondria, the cell's "energy factories." Metabolic issues that may look like FM include the following: inefficiency of energy production in the mitochondria, nutritional deficiencies (such as CoQ10, carnitine, B vitamins, magnesium, vitamin D, and others), suboptimal thyroid function, chemical and food sensitivities, reactions to medications, and other problems with body metabolism and biochemistry.

3. **Conventional medical diseases**, such as autoimmune disorders (rheumatoid arthritis, ankylosing spondylitis, lupus, multiple sclerosis, and more), Lyme disease, overt hypothyroidism, cancer, diabetes, and other illnesses.

Only in approximately one-third of cases is the person suffering from what I call classic fibromyalgia. As I mentioned in Chapter 1, classic fibromyalgia is a specific global pain syndrome that is centrally mediated, meaning that while the pain is felt everywhere, its real cause lies in the overly sensitized way the central nervous system processes ordinary stimuli. In other words, it's a kind of overreaction. This doesn't mean the pain isn't real. No, the pain is real, and it hurts. And the fatigue and other symptoms—like irritable bowel syndrome (IBS), anxiety, and depression—that often accompany fibromyalgia are also real.

But if the cause of your pain and fatigue lies in one of the other three buckets—if it's musculoskeletal, metabolic, or due to another specific medical illness—the standard treatment approach for classic FM isn't going to help you, and in some cases it may even make your symptoms worse.

And the reverse is also true. Treating someone with classic fibromyalgia for lupus or disc degeneration will not be of much help. And side effects from the wrong medications may make that person's fibromyalgia even harder to live with.

To use another analogy, suppose that Bob, Ted, Leo, and Stanley all feel feverish. They all suffer from an elevated body temperature. They all are sweating, feeling weak, and losing a healthy appetite. But Bob has an ear infection. Ted has heat stroke after a day in strong sun. Leo is having a reaction to a medication, and Stanley has the flu. Rest, lots of fluids, and a couple of aspirin may help all of them for a while, but, in each instance the root cause is different, and the treatment must also be different—just as in suspected cases of fibromyalgia.

That's why in this chapter I want to familiarize you with classic fibromyalgia and these other broad categories of conditions that "look" like fibromyalgia and also cause chronic pain, fatigue, and other typical symptoms.

Later in this chapter, you'll also answer a questionnaire that can tell you whether or not you likely suffer from classic fibromyalgia. If the answer is yes, then you should go on to read Chapter 4 to learn more about how to treat it. And if the self-test does not suggest that you have fibromyalgia, you should read the rest of the chapters in this book—especially Chapters 5, 6, and 7—to learn about the types of illnesses that masquerade as fibromyalgia syndrome. Ideally, since even people with classic fibromyalgia can have issues related to the other three buckets, as well, I recommend that everyone read all the chapters. That way, you'll get the fullest picture of the state of your health and how you can improve it.

Proper Diagnosis Is Half the Cure!

It's all too common for doctors to misdiagnose fibromyalgia and then claim that there's no known cure. That's really a double whammy: How can something you don't have be incurable? By categorizing your ailment as an incurable disease (which you may not even have) all too often the curable illness you *do* have is overlooked and treated improperly. For example, if your fatigue is caused by a chronic viral infection, like Epstein-Barr, which also causes mononucleosis, taking an antidepressant isn't going to help.

But even if you have not been misdiagnosed, even if you do have fibromyalgia, it's never true that you must learn to just live with the pain. As you'll see, there's a lot you can do to alleviate your symptoms and even retrain your central nervous system so that it perceives pain more accurately. No one with fibromyalgia is doomed to a life of pain and fatigue and a regimen of drugs for pain, depression, anxiety, and IBS. Many people with classic fibromyalgia recover completely.

Will the Real Fibromyalgia Please Stand Up?

Let's take a closer look at all four buckets, along with more detailed case histories.

Musculoskeletal Issues

One study found that of 252 people referred to a clinic for global pain treatment, 95 of them were able to find permanent relief from "widespread pain" by undertaking a course of physical therapy and other hands-on physical techniques.[3] In other words, over one-third of those studied had pain and fatigue arising not from FM but from a musculoskeletal condition such as:

- Myofascial pain syndrome (that is, referred pain from trigger points or "muscle knots")

- Musculoskeletal misalignments, postural distortions, and injuries

- Spinal joint problems, such as disc degeneration and pinched nerves

- Nerve root irritation or compression

- Tendonitis

- Injuries to the cervical spine

- Sacroiliac joint dysfunction

Arlene's Story

Arlene, a 28-year-old court stenographer, experienced pain in her shoulders, arms, and legs that kept her up at night. Unable to find a cause for her symptoms, her doctor referred her to my clinic.

Arlene led a sedentary life, hunched over a stenotype for hours at a time, without much of a life outside the courtroom. I did a number of "rule-out" tests, but they all were negative. I did note that her muscles were taut and knotted and that her body in general was stiff and in need of relaxation.

I referred Arlene to a skilled chiropractor and myofascial therapist. He concluded that she was experiencing myofascial pain, originating in a number of trigger points in her muscles. He recommended a course of myofascial therapy, which included periods of controlled compression of the trigger points, movement, stretching, and relaxation therapies. This approach made an almost immediate positive impact.

This is just one example of the type of problems that arise from a musculoskeletal issue rather than classic FM, a central nervous system disorder. The misdiagnosis of musculoskeletal issues as fibromyalgia is especially common in older patients, who may be experiencing some arthritis and fatigue that's common to their age group.

Functional Problems

Functional issues are the next bucket. Imbalances, deficiencies, and disorders in your body's metabolism can cause you to feel pain and fatigue.[4] Think of a car that runs but is misfiring, with worn spark plugs and clogged filters. It will get you there, but you'll end up paying more at the shop for the period of neglect. When areas, organs, or systems of your body aren't functioning up to par, you don't feel well, though you may not know what is off. Examples of functional disorders include:

- Suboptimal thyroid function (less obvious than the overt medical hypothyroidism)

- Mitochondrial energy metabolism dysfunction

- Adrenal exhaustion from prolonged stress

- Other subtle endocrine imbalances (in neurotransmitters, growth hormones, or other hormones)

- Dysglycemia (problems with blood sugar levels short of actual diabetes)

- Suppression or overactivation of the immune system

- Chemical and/or food sensitivities

- Reactions to medication

- Vitamin and nutrient deficiencies

- Cumulative toxic load

- Other biochemical issues, such as imbalances in bacteria and other intestinal organisms and hyper-permeability of the gut lining (called leaky gut), which can lead to more toxic metabolites entering the bloodstream, causing symptoms of chronic illness

Anne's Story

Anne was a divorced, 40-year-old systems analyst and mother of three who struggled with constant fatigue and hurt all over. She had just begun dating again and was trying to lose weight, but no matter what diet she tried—South Beach, Atkins, Paleo—she was unable to lose the pounds, while the fatigue and aching persisted. For 2 years, the practitioners she saw followed the typical combination of treatments for fibromyalgia patients: (1) medications for sleep, pain, anxiety, and/or depression; (2) mild exercise to relax the muscles and promote better bloodflow; and (3) counseling for the emotional distress.

It might have worked, except that Anne didn't have fibromyalgia— and her symptoms didn't go away. When she came to me, her lab tests confirmed my suspicion: Ann, like Judy in the earlier case, was suffering from an undiagnosed low thyroid. And when other tests came back negative, I took her off most of her other medications and put her on a daily dose of a desiccated thyroid hormone replacement. This form of complete hormone replacement contained both the thyroid hormones (T4, or thyroxine, and T3, or triiodothyronine). Anne's pain went away within a few weeks, and over the next several months, on a Paleo diet and with regular exercise, she also slowly began dropping the weight.

Other Root Causes (Conventional Medical Diseases)

In rarer instances, chronic pain and fatigue may be due to a more serious illness that has not been identified.[5] In these cases, the general recommendations in this book may not be enough to get to the root cause. You'll need to seek medical attention and undergo tests to pinpoint the nature of the issue.

In my practice, I will always order tests to rule out more serious issues. I often administer additional tests to rule out functional issues, as well. Even though I can usually ascertain classic fibromyalgia from taking a complete medical history, performing an examination, and assessing the answers to the questionnaire you will see later in this chapter, I like to confirm my diagnosis. I do this via thorough laboratory testing that rules out all other possible ailments. That testing is most essential when it comes to gaining assurance that the symptoms do not arise from a more serious disease. The questions and self-tests in this and later chapters will reveal whether that may be necessary for you. In each of the bucket chapters, I will provide information about the tests you should ask your doctor to conduct.

Let me be clear: This book is not a substitute for proper medical attention. But it will help you become both an educated consumer and your own health advocate. The information in this chapter will indicate whether it's likely that you have classic fibromyalgia. Succeeding chapters will give you a clear picture of the disorders in the three other buckets. For the majority of readers, this approach will uncover the source of their pain and fatigue. But if over the course of reading the entire book, you still don't feel clear about the nature of your condition, I recommend that you work with a doctor to find out what's going on under the hood. And I will show you how to get the best results when working with a physician.

Ryan's Story

Ryan, 45, lived in a corner of Pennsylvania surrounded by woods and old family farms. He would spend hours in his garden, producing a bountiful crop of fruits and vegetables for himself and his family. His canned tomato sauce was known throughout the valley. Almost without warning, Ryan developed pain in nearly all of his joints, making it difficult to bend or kneel. Along with the joint pain, he felt tired and depressed, and his digestion was seriously off. Instead of tying up the tomatoes, he was in a chair or in a doctor's office, trying to understand what was happening to him.

When Ryan's family doctor checked him for arthritis, the results were negative. His physician concluded that Ryan had fibromyalgia. He prescribed several medications for the pain, sleeplessness, and rumbling digestion. Still unable to work, Ryan traveled to see several specialists, and eventually came to see me. Blood tests indicated that he did have some kind of inflammation, and on further testing, it was clear that he had picked up Lyme disease, which is common enough in his region of the country. (Some of the conventional lab tests for Lyme are notoriously inaccurate and incomplete. Often more specialized and advanced testing is required to detect it.) I put him on a course of antibiotics for several weeks, as well as some other supportive therapies, and he recovered completely. By the time he got back to his garden, it was a jungle, but he—along with his neighbors—was happy he was there. And this time he was taking some extra precautions for the ticks.

Conventional diseases that can masquerade as fibromyalgia include:

- Arachnoiditis
- Cancer
- Cytomegalovirus
- Diabetes
- Epstein-Barr
- Heart and lung disease

- Iron or B-vitamin deficiency anemia
- Lyme disease
- Multiple sclerosis
- Rheumatoid arthritis
- Small fiber neuropathy

Mary's Story

Let me give you another example, this time of a more complex case involving multiple buckets that I had several years ago.

Mary had terrible digestive issues that had gone on for many years. She always felt bloated after eating and got excessively gassy, which was often a source of great embarrassment to her and affected her ability to engage in social activities she enjoyed. She described to me how sometimes after eating her stomach would distend so much it looked as if she were pregnant. Although she had dealt with digestive issues since her twenties, it was after she had had her first child, in her midthirties, that the problem got worse. At about that time, she also started to feel tremendous persistent fatigue. At first, she chalked it up to her lack of sleep and the stress that comes with attending to a young child, but it persisted even after her child got older and she was not being awakened at night by a baby.

Soon after the fatigue began, Mary also started experiencing an achiness throughout her body that never quite went away. Now she began to feel depressed and concerned about how she would take care of her family if her health was poor. When she discussed these problems with her family doctor, he did some basic blood work. And when the results came back normal, he told Mary that she needed to lower her stress and get more sleep.

The problem for Mary was that no matter how much she slept, she just never seemed to feel rejuvenated. It was always a struggle just to get out of bed once morning came—as if she hadn't slept at all. After again complaining to her family doctor, he referred her to a gastroenterologist, who performed an endoscopy and colonoscopy, which were both normal. He suggested some over-the-counter gas pills and fiber for her occasional constipation, which she had already tried. Eventually, Mary was referred to a rheumatologist who diagnosed her with fibromyalgia and put her on the medication Lyrica.

For about 2 months, Mary experienced some relief, with better sleep and a slightly better mood, but the beneficial effects of the medication waned after that, and she was soon back to feeling like she did before starting—so she stopped the medication.

Mary was beginning to feel defeated when a friend in another state told her about the success she had overcoming her chronic health problems after seeing an integrative and functional medicine doctor who was willing to take another approach. She decided to give it a try and was referred to me by another patient of mine, someone she knew through her church.

At our first meeting, we went through her entire case history, and I too wondered at first if she had FM. On the questionnaire I gave her, she marked a lot of the symptom boxes, such as achiness all around the body, persistent fatigue, unrefreshed sleep, gastrointestinal distress, and even some depression. However, she really lacked the classic history of high stress, trauma, or other problems during her childhood or in her current life. She was in a very supportive relationship with her husband and her children and had a wonderful network of friends. When I performed her physical exam, she definitely had multiple areas of pain and achiness, but it seemed that they were not just in the soft tissues but in the joints, as well. She had some muscle spasms and trigger points in larger muscle groups—including her neck, shoulders, and pelvic area—but there was definitely no hyper-perception of pain everywhere throughout the body. In fact, there were clearly many areas that elicited no pain response at all to significant pressure. This is not typical in classic FM.

We started by ordering some standard blood tests, but included many that her family doctor had not checked. We also looked at the results in a different way, with an eye toward the level of function and metabolic optimization, rather than just screening for obvious disease. Her lab tests showed the following:

☐ Markers suggestive of inflammation

☐ Autoimmune activity directed at the joint structures, including a positive rheumatoid factor

☐ An overtly normal but functionally low red blood cell count

☐ A low mean corpuscular volume (that is, her red blood cells were too small)

☐ Serum iron and ferritin (a protein that is about 20 percent iron) on the very low end of the normal range

☐ Positive thyroid peroxidase antibodies and antithyroglobulin antibodies, indicating an autoimmune disorder of the thyroid gland

☐ T3 hormone on the very low end of the normal range

Looking at these tests results, it became very clear to me that Mary didn't really have FM at all. Instead, she had a number of separate conditions that collectively appeared to add up to FM. She had some muscle problems (myofascial pain syndrome with trigger points), which placed her in the musculoskeletal bucket. She also had multiple autoimmune issues; her immune system was slowly attacking both her joints and her thyroid. She basically had early rheumatoid arthritis and Hashimoto's thyroiditis. This placed her in the other-root-causes bucket, since she actually had some well-defined medical conditions that were also contributing to her overall scenario.

While she didn't have overt anemia, meaning that her red blood cell count was still technically within a normal range, a closer look revealed that her red blood cells were in decline and their quality was diminished. The cells were too small, or what doctors call micro-cytic, making it difficult for them to carry adequate oxygen to her tissues. This is generally associated with insufficient iron levels. This was further supported by the low levels of both iron and ferritin (the storage form of iron in the body) found in the blood testing. There was no evidence of bleeding in her digestive system, and her menstrual periods were fairly typical. With this level of functional anemia, Mary could be considered to have a metabolic, or functional, problem, as well.

Finally, she did have a lot of intestinal issues without any obvi-ous GI disease. A stool analysis showed imbalances in her gastroin-testinal microflora (the microbes that live in her intestines), a condition known as dysbiosis. She also had very low output of stom-ach acid and digestive enzymes. A breath test showed a large amount of hydrogen and methane gas being produced after she consumed a specific carbohydrate intake, which supported a diag-nosis of small intestinal bacterial overgrowth (SIBO). Once again, Mary had a functional issue.

As you can see, this can all get a bit intricate, and if you aren't working with a physician or health-care provider who really under-stands these various problems and disorders, who can reason through all of the possible problems that may be causing a person's long list of symptoms, it's very easy to receive a diagnosis of FM. This is particularly true when a provider may not have the ability or experience to adequately tease out all of the subtle problems that may be ganging up on the poor person suffering from these debili-tating symptoms.

In Mary's case, we were able to address each individual problem specifically, using the methods that you'll read about in the next few chapters. Over time, she significantly improved and, ultimately, recovered. This would have never happened if she had just accepted her original incorrect diagnosis of FM and continued to take the medication she was given to treat it.

Classic Fibromyalgia

But what if your problem does not come from any of the three other buckets? What if you *do* have classic fibromyalgia?

Functional MRI scans of a person who has classic fibromyalgia show abnormal changes in pain processing in the brain itself.[6] In other words, when signals from nerve endings throughout the body reach your brain, for reasons we are just now coming to understand, the pain response is exaggerated. It's as if you called to complain that your neighbor's bachelor party had gone on too long, and the operator sent out a hook and ladder and three rescue vehicles. The response doesn't fit the stimulus. In the brain and spinal fluids of classic FM patients, researchers have found altered levels of key chemicals, including serotonin and substance P, which regulate pleasure and pain responses.

If you have fibromyalgia, you may find the oncoming lights of cars at night not just annoying but painful to look at. Or you might find yourself smiling through the agony of a pat on the back by a coworker or the affectionate embrace of an old friend. The sounds coming from the game your son and his friends are enjoying on his PlayStation may penetrate your whole body. Their squeals of delight may be felt as sharp assaults on your ears. If it's very hot or very cold, your skin may register discomfort, no matter how little or how much you are wearing. The whole world seems to have become a hostile place for you. It's not because the world has changed. Your body's perception has changed. In fibromyalgia patients, this change in perception is often triggered by a traumatic event or a series of them—a "wound" to the nervous system that causes it to become overly self-protective and on guard.

Irritable bowel syndrome is often present in true cases of fibromyalgia. Its symptoms may include constipation and/or diarrhea, distension, cramping, and bloating. To add to this unhappy picture, you may feel depressed and anxious. Your sleep, when you manage to get some, doesn't refresh you.

Stephanie's Story

At 50 years old, Stephanie had settled into a relatively happy middle age with her husband of 23 years. She had managed to escape an unhappy childhood with an abusive parent, get an education, and pursue a career she loved as a small-town lawyer. Then life threw her another challenge—sudden and persistent pain in her limbs and torso that had no apparent cause. She also felt a deep tiredness that she just could not shake. Soon thereafter, Stephanie became highly sensitive to touch. She felt stabbing pains from the tags on her blouses and other articles of clothing where they contacted her skin.

The unexplained pain and fatigue were accompanied by digestive upsets, making it difficult for Stephanie to know what to eat. When she arrived at my clinic and I took a patient history, I learned that her symptoms appeared after two recent events. First, her mother had died at 95. And in the aftermath, her sister revealed childhood memories of being molested by their father.

Stephanie felt that her own symptoms were psychosomatic—an interpretation that her therapist supported enthusiastically. Worst of all, she felt guilty that she could be of so little support to her sister.

Was Stephanie suffering from classic fibromyalgia?

To me, it seemed highly possible from her patient history. It's well established that experiencing extreme stress during childhood (when the nervous system and its responses are developing) can alter the way that people deal with stress and perceive their world. Young girls are more vulnerable, particularly if they feel unsafe at home or abandoned or betrayed by those who are responsible for protecting them. Verbal abuse, physical abuse, and, most seriously, sexual abuse, can literally shatter the nervous system and change the limbic system, an area of the brain often called the emotional brain.

I ran a number of tests on Stephanie and did a hands-on examination. The exam showed no tissue injury or structural problems. The tests all came up negative. I began treating Stephanie for fibromyalgia with detox, diet, careful supplementation, relaxation, and very light self-massage. I also persuaded her to cut back on the four cups of coffee she was drinking every day and the glass of California cabernet sauvignon she consumed every night at dinner, which for her was a form of self-medication.

Instead, to help her wind down and get to sleep, I gave her the muscle-relaxant mineral magnesium. And working with her therapist, who had by now acknowledged there was a physiological issue, I prescribed a low-dose SNRI (serotonin and norepinephrine reuptake inhibitor) antidepressant medication and key neurotransmitter precursor nutrients. After a few weeks on this regimen, Stephanie started to feel normal again. She also felt more refreshed from sleep. Her extreme sensitivity was greatly diminished, and she was able to be present for her family in ways she hadn't been for months.

The Fibromyalgia Clinical Reasoning Guide

The graphic in Figure 3.1 is a kind of visual summary of the four buckets and the symptoms usually associated with each. Along with the stories you have just read, this visual may help you get a clearer picture of how either classic fibromyalgia or the three forms of pseudo-fibromyalgia (that is, false fibromyalgia, meaning it is really something else) can cause symptoms of chronic pain and fatigue.

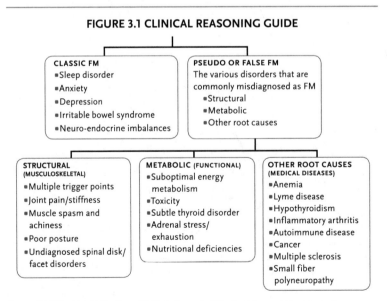

FIGURE 3.1 CLINICAL REASONING GUIDE

CLASSIC FM
- Sleep disorder
- Anxiety
- Depression
- Irritable bowel syndrome
- Neuro-endocrine imbalances

PSEUDO OR FALSE FM
The various disorders that are commonly misdiagnosed as FM
- Structural
- Metabolic
- Other root causes

STRUCTURAL (MUSCULOSKELETAL)
- Multiple trigger points
- Joint pain/stiffness
- Muscle spasm and achiness
- Poor posture
- Undiagnosed spinal disk/facet disorders

METABOLIC (FUNCTIONAL)
- Suboptimal energy metabolism
- Toxicity
- Subtle thyroid disorder
- Adrenal stress/exhaustion
- Nutritional deficiencies

OTHER ROOT CAUSES (MEDICAL DISEASES)
- Anemia
- Lyme disease
- Hypothyroidism
- Inflammatory arthritis
- Autoimmune disease
- Cancer
- Multiple sclerosis
- Small fiber polyneuropathy

Source: M. Schneider, D. Brady, and S. Perle, Journal of Manipulative and Physiological Therapeutics 29 (2006): 495–501. Used with permission.

Do You Have Classic Fibromyalgia?

Below you'll find the questionnaire previously mentioned. Answering these five questions will reveal whether it's likely that you have classic fibromyalgia—or not. Note the word *likely*, since a definitive answer may require a doctor's visit and some further testing. But this initial test, originating with the American College of Rheumatology's most recent diagnostic criteria, while far from perfect, is the current gold standard for diagnosing FM. It can spare you a lot of time and energy traveling down fruitless pathways. This is because, while there are many illnesses that masquerade as fibromyalgia, there are certain markers that are unmistakable signs of FM, and the test will look for these. If the test

---

FIGURE 3.2 FIBROMYALGIA QUESTIONNAIRE

A. Over the past week (7-days) indicate below if you have had achiness/tenderness/pain in the areas indicated in the body diagrams. (Add up all locations with pain, assigning the number 1 for each location. Total possible points equal 19).

TOTAL SCORE: _____

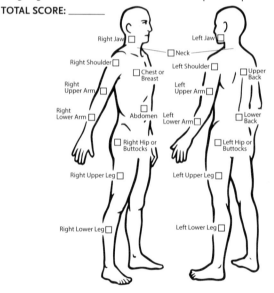

B. Indicate the level of the three symptoms listed below that you have experienced over the past week (7 days), using the scale provided.

	Not present/ No problem	Mild or occasional problem	Moderate and persistent problem	Severe and continuous problem
Points	0	1	2	3
Fatigue:	☐	☐	☐	☐
Unrefreshed sleep:	☐	☐	☐	☐
Brain fog/memory problems:	☐	☐	☐	☐

TOTAL SCORE: _____

suggests that you have FM, pay close attention to the information and instructions in Chapter 4, which will help you understand classic fibromyalgia and the best options for successfully managing it.

If the questionnaire suggests you do not have classic fibromyalgia, continue to read Chapters 5, 6, and 7 to see which of the other categories of pseudo-fibromyalgia your symptoms most likely belong in.

Take the test in Figure 3.2 now. It might be easier to make a photocopy of the test first. You can also go to FibroFix.com to download a copy. Answer the questions to the best of your ability based on what you know about your health history at this time.

C. Indicate if you have experienced the following symptoms listed below. Place "0" as your score if you have not experienced the symptom and a "1" if you have experienced the symptom over the past 6 months.

- Irritable bowel (pain, cramping, gas, diarrhea, constipation, etc.): _____
- Depression and/or anxiety: _____
- Headache: _____
  TOTAL SCORE: _____

D. Answer "yes" or "no" to the following two questions:

    a. Have any symptoms listed as present in   □ Yes   □ No
       sections B and C been present and fairly
       consistent in severity over the past 3 months?

    b. Have you been diagnosed with any medical   □ Yes   □ No
       condition or disease that may be the cause of
       your symptoms and complaints?

SCORING AND INTERPRETATION:

Add your total numerical scores from sections A, B, and C:
GRAND TOTAL SCORE: _____

To be consistent with the diagnostic criteria for a diagnosis of "classic" fibromyalgia, you must at a minimum have:

    1. A grand total score of 13 or greater (total possible points = 31).
    2. You must have answered "yes" to question D (a) and "no" to question D (b).

YOUR RESULTS: Using the scoring and interpretation of the criteria above, is your overall result indicative of likely classic fibromyalgia? (Circle one below).

YES or NO

Source: Based on the 2011 Modification of the American College of Rheumatology Preliminary Diagnostic Criteria for Fibromyalgia.

How to Score the Test

A total score of 12 or less on questions 1, 2, and 3 suggests that you probably do not have fibromyalgia. It's highly unusual for someone with a score that low to have classic FM. On the other hand, a score of 13 or greater is consistent with a possible diagnosis of fibromyalgia. But there's one important caveat: Question 4 must be answered "yes" and question 5 must be answered "no." That is, you must have had your symptoms for at least 3 months, and there must not be any other disorder present that can otherwise explain your pain. I advise that you work with a doctor, or other health-care provider, who is fully familiar with FM to help determine the accurate answer to question 5.

In addition, along with a score of 13 or above and "yes" and "no" answers on questions 4 and 5, respectively, you must be experiencing at least two of these symptoms:

- Anxiety

- Depression

- Nonrefreshing sleep

- Irritable bowel syndrome (usually with constipation and/or diarrhea, cramping, bloating, and distension)

If you don't have at least two of the above symptoms, even though you have body achiness and fatigue, then the source of your problems is probably *not* classic FM. Your issues are very likely *not* centrally mediated by the nervous system.

To summarize, it's likely that you have classic fibromyalgia if:

- You have a total score of 13 or above on questions 1, 2, and 3 of the questionnaire

- You answered "yes" to question 4 and "no" to question 5

- You have at least two of the symptoms mentioned in the list above

If you did not "pass" the test, I'm not saying you don't hurt, only that you're probably not in the classic bucket. In Chapters 5, 6, and 7, I'm going to walk you through the other buckets, step by step. In those chapters, you'll find tests and questionnaires for metabolic and musculoskeletal issues to help you draw closer to pinpointing the source of your discomfort. Ultimately, it's always advisable for you to have a comprehensive examination and workup by a physician competent in FM to con-firm that you do not have some other medical condition that could be causing your symptoms. You'll learn more about how you can work with your health-care provider to definitively rule out other medical condi-tions in Chapter 7.

Other Resources

As you start to narrow down the source of your symptoms, you'll find resources at the end of this book for locating physicians who know how to take the right kind of in-depth patient history, conduct a thorough physical examination, and run various useful tests that I will recom-mend. If you wish to, you can take this book along with its lists of tests and discuss them with your doctor. Lab testing can help to determine key neurotransmitter levels, blood cell counts, mitochondrial energy pro-duction, adrenal function, and stress response as well as the presence of Lyme, anemia, a malignancy, thyroid and autoimmune disorders, and many more, all of which can be in play with chronic pain and fatigue.

Conclusion

In this chapter, you discovered—by understanding your symptoms, answering the questionnaires, and learning how to work with your doctor—whether you likely have classic fibromyalgia or one of the ill-nesses that often masquerades as fibromyalgia.

In the next four chapters, I examine classic fibromyalgia and its chief imposters. These chapters will also focus on practical steps you can take to work with these illnesses.

If you are not sure of the source of your chronic pain and fatigue, read on. But even if you think you know your diagnosis now, I advise you to read all these chapters. As I have mentioned, those who suffer from global pain may be dealing with more than one condition, and these chapters contain valuable information.

Whether you're seeking to diagnose and work with your health issues or looking for the right kind of medical testing, this book will help you understand and eliminate your chronic pain and fatigue.

CHAPTER 4

THE CLASSIC FIBROMYALGIA FIX

I f you are reading this chapter, it may be because you think (based on the questionnaire you took in the last chapter) that you are one of the approximately 20 percent of chronic pain sufferers who actually have classic fibromyalgia.

Classic fibromyalgia is a difficult and painful illness. But diagnosing it is more than half the battle. It's by no means the life sentence that many people have been warned about by their doctors. Once you understand what you are dealing with (and what you aren't dealing with), there are many avenues of relief, and in some cases, your fibromyalgia may disappear altogether. In fact, the multipronged approach I recommend in this chapter can bring relief within weeks and a more dramatic restoration of health within a few months.

But please understand that there's no quick fix or single treatment for classic fibromyalgia. In most cases, a person with classic FM is dealing with a combination of problems requiring a combination of solutions.

A Multifaceted Approach

Because the illness is multifaceted, the treatment approach has to be, too. Let's review some of the common symptoms of classic FM.

- Widespread pain/tenderness

- Extreme fatigue/low energy

- Nonrefreshing sleep

- Difficulty concentrating

- Inability to tolerate exercise

- Irritable bowel syndrome (constipation and/or diarrhea, bloating, distension, and cramping)

- History of depression/anxiety

- Irritable bladder syndrome

- Small intestinal bacterial overgrowth (SIBO)

- Extreme sensitivity to touch

- Migraine headaches

- Grinding/clenching teeth

- Multiple chemical/food sensitivities

Of course, you probably don't have all of these issues, and you may have one or two others that are not listed here. You may very likely have some muscle and joint problems as well as some metabolic issues that are compounding your classic FM pain. And because the underlying cause of classic FM is often related to emotional stress or previous traumatic experiences, the most effective treatment is a combination approach that looks at those issues, as well.

To be absolutely certain of what's going on, I always recommend getting some additional tests. A qualified functional medicine doctor can also perform a physical exam that will help to confirm what you learned about your pain syndrome in Chapter 3. All the tests that I advise you to speak to your doctor or health-care practitioner about can be found in the Additional Resources section of this book (page 259).

If this book (and consultation with your doctor) helps you determine that you have classic FM, understand that it's a real problem with a real solution. But there's no quick fix or single treatment.

In addition to using the diet, movement, and mind-body approaches on the Fibro-Fix Foundational Plan, I treat classic fibromyalgia by introducing supports that encourage the body's own healing and resetting the nervous system's response to stress and pain. I'll also consider medications that aim to help with global pain, fatigue, and other symptoms, which I'll tell you about later in this chapter. Unfortunately, these medications often have unwanted side effects. And taken alone, without other modes of treatment, they have another drawback: By sometimes successfully masking your symptoms, they can delay or prevent you from dealing with the root cause of your FM. That is why I prescribe natural supplements and specific treatments whenever possible and resort to medications only when they are absolutely appropriate and necessary.

The Fibro-Fix Foundational Plan (Chapter 2) is an excellent start. The plan reduces general inflammation, removes allergens from your diet, gives you lots of protein as you detox, and introduces some mild mobility exercises. But the plan is designed as an overall approach to use before the precise cause of your global pain and fatigue has been discovered. Once you know for certain that you are dealing with classic fibromyalgia, we add the following to address conditions unique to this illness.

- Support for serotonin levels to help with pain, unrefreshing sleep, emotional stress, depression, and irritable bowel syndrome

- Medications and herbal supplements for sleep, pain, stress, anxiety, and depression

- Psychological counseling for dealing with and reducing prior emotional distress that may be associated with fibromyalgia

This is the approach that I believe any doctor who understands fibromyalgia should take.

Molly's Story

When Molly dragged herself into my office early one spring day, I recognized the worry, depression, and exhaustion that frequently dog people with classic FM. I ordered some basic tests to rule out diseases that might mimic FM symptoms, but the tests came back negative. That's when I performed a comprehensive hands-on physical examination and gave her the questionnaires I use to probe more deeply. After ruling out other problems, I was able to confirm a classic FM diagnosis. In addition to pain, Molly also suffered from the anxiety and poor sleep so common to FM.

Molly was trapped in a vicious cycle. Her hypersensitive nervous system made being awake a kind of living nightmare. Whatever she touched, or touched her, caused her pain. In short order, the world had become a hostile place, and she moved through it cautiously and fearfully, like someone walking on thin ice. And while Molly's days were suddenly fraught with new dangers, the nights were no relief, for she could not sleep. Instead, she lay on the bed anxious about her condition—and anxious about her anxiety. In the morning, with only a few hours at most of actual sleep, she awoke unrefreshed, her nervous system even less prepared than it was the day before for the raw encounters she would have with the people and objects around her.

To start, I suggested that Molly take sustained-released melatonin, a natural sleep aid, before bedtime, along with a natural serotonin enhancer to help reduce her anxiety, improve the quality of her sleep, and positively alter her pain perception. We will revisit her story soon. But first I want to explore with you the mechanism of classic fibromyalgia.

What's Going on in Your Body?

What kinds of imbalances exist in the bodies of those with classic fibromyalgia? And why do these imbalances occur?

Although the specific cause of classic FM is unknown, our best estimation is that it usually originates early in life due to emotional or physical stress or trauma. The still-developing nervous system reacts strongly to traumatic experiences, such as a severe car accident, an injury, a surgical procedure, or physical or emotional abuse. Even *witnessing* a horrific event at an early age can lead to the neurological response pattern underlying FM. Physical or emotional traumas that happen later in life do not commonly cause classic fibromyalgia, though in someone who has had earlier traumas, they may be the straw that breaks the camel's back, so to speak, and trigger its onset.

To give you an idea of the kinds of incidents that may be troubling, I have adapted the following questionnaire, developed by Dr. J Douglas Brennar at Emory University. You don't have to answer the questionnaire or ponder it extensively. Just read through it to get an idea of past experiences that may have contributed to your developing FM.

EARLY TRAUMA SELF-REPORT FORM

General Traumas	Yes	No
Were you ever exposed to a life-threatening natural disaster?	Yes	No
Were you ever involved in a serious car accident?	Yes	No
Did you ever suffer a serious personal injury or illness?	Yes	No
Did you ever experience the death of a parent or primary caretaker?	Yes	No
Did you ever experience the death or serious injury of a friend?	Yes	No
Did you ever witness violence toward others, including family members?	Yes	No
Has anyone in your family suffered from a mental or psychiatric illness or suffered a mental "breakdown"?	Yes	No
Did your parents or primary caretaker have a problem with alcoholism or drug abuse?	Yes	No
Did you ever see someone murdered?	Yes	No
Physical Punishment		
Were you ever slapped in the face with an open hand?	Yes	No
Were you ever deliberately burned by hot water, a cigarette, or something else?	Yes	No
Were you ever punched or kicked?	Yes	No
Were you ever hit with an object that was thrown at you?	Yes	No
Were you ever pushed or shoved?	Yes	No
Emotional Abuse		
Were you often put down or ridiculed?	Yes	No
Were you often ignored or made to feel that you didn't count?	Yes	No
Were you often told you were no good?	Yes	No
Most of the time, were you treated in a cold, uncaring way and made to feel you were not loved?	Yes	No
Did your parents or caretakers often fail to understand you or your needs?	Yes	No
Sexual Events		
Were you ever touched in an intimate or private part of your body (e.g., breast, thighs, genitals) in a way that surprised you or made you feel uncomfortable?	Yes	No
Did you ever experience someone rubbing his or her genitals against you?	Yes	No
Were you ever forced to touch a person in an intimate or private part of his or her body?	Yes	No
Did anyone ever have genital sex with you against your will?	Yes	No
Were you ever forced to kiss someone in a sexual rather than an affectionate way?	Yes	No

(continued)

If you responded "Yes" to any of the above events, answer the following questions for the one that has had the greatest impact on your life. When answering, consider how you felt at the time of the event.

Did you experience emotions of intense fear, horror, or helplessness?		Yes	No
Did you feel out-of-your-body or as if you were in a dream?		Yes	No

Adapted from the Early Trauma Inventory Self Report-Short Form (ETISR-SF), J. Douglas Bremner, Emory University School of Medicine, Atlanta, GA. Used with permission.

Note: While there is no formal scoring system that I recommend pertaining to this questionnaire that definitively determines if you are suffering from classic FM or not, the more you answered "yes," the more consistent your early life history is with the development of FM in later life.

When young children with developing nervous systems experience any of the emotional, physical, or sexual traumas defined in the questionnaire, the prolonged stress that results can start to confuse their central nervous systems into overresponding to stimuli. As a result, nerve signals "widen" or "spill over" onto other neurons (neuroscientists call this a widening of the receptive fields of pain), such that the central nervous system misinterprets an array of harmless stimuli as painful or threatening. This also results in stimuli that should *not* cause pain, such as light touch, being interpreted as pain in an ever-expanding area of your body, instead of just where the touch emanated. In a sense, you could say that the original trauma continues to reverberate through your nervous system, even when nothing that would ordinarily cause pain is present. Once triggered, this hypersensitivity may extend into an emotional and physical pain syndrome.

Let's revisit Molly's story. She had been experiencing severe fatigue along with widespread pain for over 2 years. When I probed further, I found out that her symptoms had noticeably worsened at the time her husband lost his job. During that period, she also began having panic attacks. Moreover, in talking further with Molly about her past, I learned that as a child she had been in an automobile crash that killed her older brother.

This was the "aha" moment that reconfirmed my diagnosis. It also gave Molly a new understanding about what I was asking her to do. With her newfound confidence, Molly began the Fibro-Fix Foundational Plan and followed it up with treatments we will discuss later in this chapter. Soon she was ready to begin using the right supplements and stress management techniques to support her recovery. All of the approaches worked together to send her nervous system new messages to dial down her stress, calm her perception of pain, and reduce her other symptoms.

In this book, I offer physical supports to help your nervous system readjust. I also recommend cognitive behavioral therapy, including guided imagery, for reorienting your neurological responses.

The Importance of Serotonin

It was once thought that our brains and nervous systems were like an electrical wiring grid, but research now tells us that they are much more complicated than this. The brain and nervous system may be more like a complex hologram than a simple electrical schematic.

Many chemicals are involved in the transmission of nerve impulses, messages, and the other complicated functions of the nervous system. Our nerve cells, or neurons, aren't a continuous "wire." Rather, there are gaps, called synapses, between them. Neurotransmitters are the chemicals that carry the nerve signals across those gaps. And once they have

NEW APPROACHES TO TRAUMA

Since September 11, 2001, our understanding of how to best treat trauma has changed. While it's helpful to *identify* traumas or stresses that were triggering, as you have done in looking over the questionnaire, there are other approaches once thought to be helpful that I would not recommend. For example, recalling and talking extensively about these past experiences is now considered less helpful than previously thought. Why? Because while insight may be gained, repeatedly recalling the trauma actually reactivates the very neurological responses that the therapies I offer here aim to calm. This is in line with a new movement in counseling, called forgiveness therapy, that supports greater acceptance of past traumas and even trying to forgive the perpetrator of the abuse. This approach has been very helpful to some, without having the person relive the traumatizing event over and over again.[1]

carried a signal from one neuron to another, they are either reabsorbed back into the neuron that initially released them (a process known as reuptake) or metabolized by enzymes. Not all neurotransmitters are involved in helping electrical signals pass from neuron to neuron, though. Others are used to signal some other physiological response, such as secretion of a hormone or other chemical messenger. It can all get very complicated indeed, with a virtual cascade of chemicals and resulting physiological changes and effects. We still aren't even close to fully understanding the complicated workings of the nervous system.

For FM, probably the most important neurotransmitter is serotonin. Serotonin is the "mood chemical" that produces feelings of well-being and happiness. It also helps regulate appetite, sleep, and, yes, pain perception. It was low serotonin levels that contributed to the anxiety and sleeplessness that Molly suffered from.

As we've seen, sleep is vitally important, because if you don't get adequate rest, then the body simply does not have the opportunity to repair itself, resulting in more stress on all the tissues and organs of the body. This includes the brain and nervous system. This lack of repair and rest results in dysfunction of that tissue or organ, and it also causes you to feel profound, unrelenting fatigue.

Substance P

In classic FM, serotonin levels are low in both the central nervous system and the cerebral spinal fluid (CSF), the fluid which bathes the spinal cord. And when serotonin levels are low, levels of another neurotransmitter called substance P tend to be high. Substance P is also a neuromodulator involved in determining pain levels. Substance P can be released from the sensory nerve fibers in your skin, muscles, joints, and spinal cord. Because it's so ubiquitous, when there's too much substance P, a pain signal can "widen" or "spill over" onto other neurons that are not part of the initial stimulus, enhancing and spreading the pain. This is similar to a referred pain, one that originates in one area but is also felt in another. In addition to governing the level of substance P, serotonin governs something called the descending antinociceptive system, or DANS, which I call the pain gate manager.

The Pain Gate Manager

The DANS pain gate manager is a pathway in the spinal cord that dampens the sensation of pain. Just as painful stimuli open what neurologists call "the pain gate," it's the job of DANS to close it.

Here's an example of how this works in your body every day. Remember what it feels like to wear a shirt. Your body "knows" that you have a shirt on because you feel it on your skin. Within a few minutes of putting on your shirt, the pain gate manager correctly interprets that it's just a shirt and poses no danger to your body. It's useless information that the pain gate manager shuts off, and you no longer sense that you have a shirt on all throughout the day. As with other nearly automatic bodily mechanisms, your body adjusts. (Figure 4.1 shows the DANS process in detail.)

FIGURE 4.1 THE DESCENDING ANTINOCICEPTIVE SYSTEM

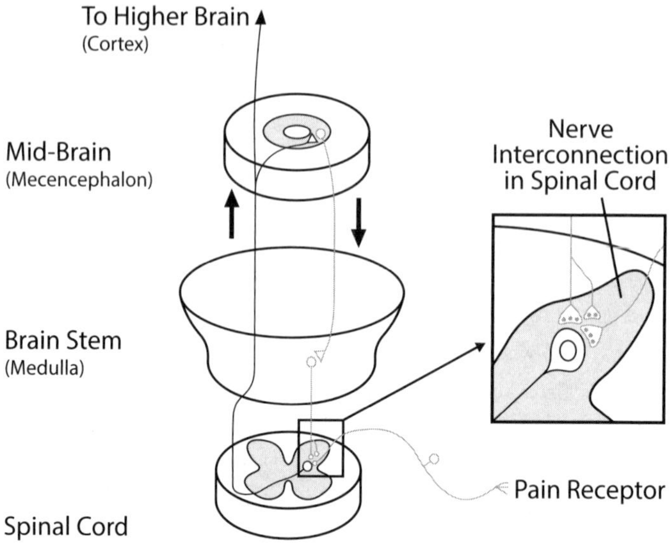

To Higher Brain
(Cortex)

Mid-Brain
(Mecencephalon)

Nerve
Interconnection
in Spinal Cord

Brain Stem
(Medulla)

Spinal Cord

Pain Receptor

But if serotonin levels are low and substance P is high, the gates open wide. As a result, not only does your sensory perception widen but DANS' ability to close the gate is also blunted. This can result in feeling pain from even slight contact with your shirt, or from a light touch. In other words, the pain gate manager can no longer manage pain effectively. This produces one of the hallmark symptoms of classic fibromyalgia—a lowered pain threshold.

The initial changes in the nervous system that ultimately produce this lower pain threshold, and most of the associated symptoms of classic FM, probably occur in the limbic system—commonly referred to as the emotional center of the brain. The limbic system has far-reaching effects on many other body systems, including the hypothalamic-pituitary-adrenal axis (which controls your stress response), the sympathetic and parasympathetic nervous systems, and the descending anti-nociceptive system.

Serotonin and Irritable Bowel Syndrome

Serotonin has yet another role to play in classic FM. It is the main messenger molecule for the part of your nervous system that controls the intestinal tract and governs digestion, the enteric nervous system. Low serotonin levels therefore interfere with the proper functioning of your digestive system. The result is that people with FM very frequently also suffer from irritable bowel syndrome (IBS) and the discomfort that comes along with it. Another way of stating this is that a dysfunction involving serotonin, when it occurs in the central nervous system, can result in FM, but when it occurs in the enteric nervous system, it results in IBS. This is why, in my experience, the vast majority of those with FM also have IBS.

The primary symptoms of IBS are abdominal pain and a change in bowel habits, such as diarrhea or constipation. There may also be a sense of urgency around bowel movements, feelings of incomplete evacuation, and bloating. Very commonly, people with IBS may have gastroesophageal reflux, chronic fatigue syndrome, fibromyalgia, headache, backache, depression, and anxiety. Sexual dysfunction is also common with irritable bowel syndrome. (IBS will be discussed in greater detail in Chapter 6, page 166.)

Cleo's Story

Along with her classic FM, Cleo had very uncomfortable gut issues—typical of irritable bowel syndrome. It was difficult for her to know what was okay to eat because so many foods appeared to cause a reaction. As sometimes occurs, the onset of her gut problems preceded the other more classic FM symptoms. Cleo's gut problems began after her long-time boss was forced into early retirement. His replacement was a fast-talking and ambitious younger woman who one-by-one targeted the firm's long-term employees, finding excuses to fire them. For a period of 6 months, Cleo sensed that she would be next, and eventually that turned out to be the case. But even before she got her pink slip, her gut reacted to the stress of her struggle to keep her job. With the FM and the IBS, Cleo had withdrawn from most of the activities that she had previously enjoyed. She was afraid to leave home in the event that she might have a gut "episode," a sudden onset of diarrhea.

I placed Cleo on the Fibro-Fix Foundational Plan. Removing key inflammatory foods, and foods she was likely sensitive to, was helpful. Her gut problems lessened slightly. Next, with my encouragement, she began to take a short daily walk in a nearby wooded area. This helped release the stress she had carried from her former workplace.

Treating Low Serotonin

From all that you have just read, you should now understand why one of the main goals of treating classic fibromyalgia is raising serotonin levels. The question is, how best to do it? Before I go on to reveal the treatments that helped Molly and many others, let me first explain why supplements are so crucial to successful treatment—for FM, for other pain syndromes, and for a wide range of chronic ailments.

The Importance of Supplements

For decades, conventional Western medicine has downplayed the importance of vitamins and supplements. Instead, it has invested its efforts and money in the drug model of health care. Medicine is a very territorial and financially driven business, and the vitamin issue is as much a turf, market-share, and money battle as it is anything else. That is why medical authorities often state that people do not need to concern themselves with supplemental vitamin pills. While it's true that there are many examples of hype regarding supplements, there's also a plethora of positive evidence across a wide span of applications.

You may even hear that vitamins are a waste of money and that anyone advocating their use is a quack or a snake-oil salesman. The implication is that all the vitamins and minerals you could ever need are in the food you eat, particularly if you live in a wealthy Western country where food is plentiful. This all *sounds* logical. But it rests on the doubtful assumption that the average person eats fresh, unprocessed, healthy, whole food at every meal. If that were true, vitamin pills really would not be necessary. Unfortunately, many Americans, and people in other Western industrialized countries, consume—or subsist entirely on—unhealthy foods. Our food is all too often processed and full of sweeteners, allergens, toxic chemicals, and pesticides and devoid of vitamins and minerals.

The Essential Role of Vitamins and Minerals

Vitamins and minerals are micronutrients that act as catalysts for the enzymes that perform necessary biochemical activity in our bodies. When micronutrient levels are too low, your biochemistry and metabolism will not function optimally. This can lead to fatigue, depression, and in some cases even disease. And there's no standard that applies to every individual. For example, the so-called average American is not a real person but rather an arbitrary, mathematical construct. Who is average? Some people need more of a particular vitamin or mineral in order to drive a particular enzyme harder. And due to genetic differences, some of us may not make optimal amounts of this or that particular enzyme. Or we may make a slightly incorrect version of that enzyme. Often, people with FM need more of certain key nutrients because of the alterations in their stress response due to early stress and trauma.

When you look at how much chemically laden, calorie-rich, nutrient-poor processed foods have become a part of our daily diets, the concept of supplementing with vitamins and minerals is not so radical at all. Were humans meant to take vitamin pills? No more than we were designed to consume Big Macs, Coca-Cola, and margarine!

The First Supplements

Originally, the concept of supplementing food to make up for nutrient deficiencies came not from standard medical doctors but from the public health arena. An example of this is adding iodine to table salt. Before this was done, goiters were fairly common in the United States, particularly in the northern Midwestern states. In fact, this region of the United States used to be referred to as the Goiter Belt. That is because the soil there is iodine deficient, and at a time when most foods were locally grown, this meant that people's diets were as well. So a decision was made to add iodine to something that was consumed on a regular basis—like table salt.

A similar decision was made to add B vitamins to white bread, since refining, bleaching, and processing wheat depletes it of its vitamin and mineral content, leaving not much more than calories behind. Although almost 30 nutrients are depleted during wheat processing, the government requires manufacturers to put back only about eight. Based on this addition of nutrients, the somewhat ironic phrase "enriched white bread" was coined.

More and more scientific data is emerging that suggests nutritional deficiencies are becoming rampant as we consume more devitalized and processed foods. In fact, behavioral difficulties in our children and violent behaviors in adults have been linked to nutritional deficiencies. Public health officials have won a few battles over adding certain nutrients to our foods, but unfortunately that has only happened in more serious situations.

The Bias against Supplements

The orthodox medical establishment generally continues to fiercely criticize supplementation. Positive studies on micronutrients are often picked apart, while negative ones are run up the flagpole as triumphs. When the media reports positive results, the findings are characterized as "new discoveries" even though, in many cases, open-minded physicians have been recommending these scientifically validated supplements for decades. In other words, the medical establishment takes the position that the vitamin doesn't work unless we are ready to say it does and can claim credit for the finding.

Besides, why take the time to educate your patient about healthy nutrition when you can write a prescription for a drug in less than 1 minute? In the 6 to 10 minutes that the fast-paced and high-volume modern medical practice model allows a doctor to see a patient, there's no time to talk about diet. Doctors also are generally taught that diet doesn't matter much—despite the research refuting this—since the answer for most symptoms lies in medication. These aren't bad people;

they are just indoctrinated this way in their conventional training.

However, doctors are also very smart people or they would not have gotten into medical school in the first place. They remember being taught about the function of vitamins and minerals as key regulators of biochemistry in their premedical studies, but then in medical school that knowledge was discounted in favor of lucrative drug-based therapies, where all of the money is generated in modern medicine. Many of them figure this out at some point and get frustrated with the realities of conventional medical practice. This is why so many physicians are going back to school or attending postgraduate education conferences, to learn more about the use of therapeutic nutrition—including the strategic use of dietary changes, vitamins, minerals, and herbal or botanical supplements—along with proper movement and exercise and various stress management techniques.

Along with a handful of vanguard doctors, it's the public who demanded that vitamins and minerals be investigated further. And there's more and more scientific evidence every day that vitamins and minerals play a large role in wellness and can actually be used therapeutically to effectively and inexpensively treat certain diseases. One study using Medicare data from individuals over 65 years old indicated that the use of a daily multivitamin over a 5-year period could prevent $3.9 billion in Medicare payments, even after paying for the supplements, a net savings of $1.6 billion.[2]

VITAMIN E AND HEART DISEASE

Examples of some of the under- and improperly reported effects of vitamins on health can be illustrated with vitamin E and heart disease. Heart disease is the number one killer in our society, and long-standing scientific evidence clearly shows that vitamin E can help in its prevention. Recently, two studies implied that vitamin E might actually be dangerous and lead to increased deaths. But on closer inspection, what these studies actually showed is that the long-term use of *synthetic* vitamin E can be problematic. The natural mixture of vitamin E—found in foods like nuts, seeds, green leafy vegetables, and oily fish and in quality, mixed-form vitamin E supplements—has a long established history of safely preventing disease.[3]

This is an example of how one improperly or incompletely reported study can mislead people—though in this case, there are many more positive studies than negative ones. For instance, another study showed that supplementation with 400 IU of vitamin E per day reduced the incidence of heart attacks by 77 percent.[4] And an 8-year study on over 87,000 nurses showed that supplementation with 200 IU of vitamin E for 2 years or more resulted in a 41 percent reduction in cardiovascular disease.[5] The Health Professionals Follow-Up Study, a study on almost 40,000 men, revealed a 37 percent reduction in cardiovascular disease in those subjects consuming at least 400 IU of vitamin E per day.[6] If a new pharmaceutical drug produced results such as these, the media attention these findings would command would be staggering. Why are the public and their physicians virtually unaware of this information?

Because this kind of bias has gone on for so long, it would be professional suicide for orthodox medicine to suddenly do an about-face and admit that they were wrong all along. That would mean a loss of professional clout, credibility, and cultural authority. If a profession loses credibility, the loss often translates into a loss of market share and money. In fact, nearly two decades ago, in 1997, office visits to nonconventional health-care providers outnumbered those to conventional primary care physicians for the first time in the United States. Therein lies the turf battle.

How the Prescription Drug Market Really Works

It's no secret that the big money that drives medicine is made by the development and sale of proprietary prescription drugs. The goal of this game is to develop a drug and patent it. If granted a patent, the developing company has the right to manufacture and market that drug, without competition, for a 12-year period to offset the money spent researching and developing it. During this time, the newly patented drug can be sold for as much as the market will bear. In the past decade, Medicare reform legislation containing prescription drug coverage was finally passed, but drug company lobbyists were able to successfully work into the new law a provision that the US government could not even negotiate drug prices. That is right. You read it correctly. The biggest customer of the pharmaceutical industry was legally prohibited from negotiating a better price for medications purchased in massive quantities. Can you imagine this occurring in any other industry? With new health-care reform, the US Congress has been trying to make changes to this policy.

Note also that, generally, in order for a company to be granted a patent, the substance must be *man-made*. It can't occur naturally. If the substance can be found in nature, then nobody can own it, and it's therefore ineligible for a proprietary patent. The majority of the time, drugs originate from some plant or natural material with a known therapeutic application that is then chemically modified just enough to make it a *synthetic* compound that is eligible for patent. This process often results in a substance that is more potent per dose and faster acting but also one that may possess significant side effects. The toxins produced by the drug have to be rendered harmless and eliminated by the liver and kidneys, which requires large amounts of vitamins and minerals that function as part of the detoxification system.

The Question of Research

An argument I hear often from conventional-minded physicians is that there's not enough research to support the use of vitamins, minerals, herbs, and other natural supplements. While the government helps fund staggering amounts of drug-based research and the deep pockets of the pharmaceutical industry contributes even more, how much research money is funneled to the study of vitamins, herbs, and other natural agents? The answer is, not much, or now—due to political and market pressures—a token amount. From a research perspective, it's simply not a fair fight. In my experience, many physicians do not look at the substantial amount of research that actually exists on the use of these natural compounds before stating that there's none. It is really frustrating indeed. In the end, it's quite simple. What is good for the pharmaceutical industry is good for organized, conventional medicine as we know it today. This is the industry that fuels the machine.

Medical school students are generally taught, whether overtly or subtly, that drugs and surgery are the only ways to treat the majority of ailments and that anything else is just not serious medicine. Is that any surprise when they may have had their classes in the Pfizer wing of their medical school? This mind-set continues throughout doctors' careers as pharmaceutical sales reps visit their offices with the goal of convincing them to use the newest drugs. I have personally observed drug salespeople telling doctors to use the new drug with the fresh 12-year patent, since the older drug coming off patent *really didn't work as well as the new one anyway and had lots more side effects.* What about the previous 12 years when those same drug salespeople were telling the doctors that the old drug was the best thing since sliced bread, had little or no side effects, and was the perfect solution for a particular problem? You need to understand that when a drug patent runs out other manufacturers can then make a generic form of the drug and offer it to the market at a much lower cost. That is why it's advantageous for a pharmaceutical company to have a new drug ready when its older drug's protective patent is about to expire.

Unfortunately, the majority of physicians receive a great deal of their postdoctoral pharmacological education from these drug company sales representatives. In fact, it has been suggested by some that the majority of information absorbed by doctors while reading medical journals is from the advertisements, not the technical articles, and that the advertisements in medical journals are not entirely evidence-based. What do you think is being advertised in medical journals anyway? You guessed it, drugs.

Of course, on the other hand, some proponents of vitamins and nutritional supplements make some pretty bold claims about vitamin therapy that are not firmly supported by the scientific literature. These situations should be condemned to the same degree. I often encourage doctors, and patients alike, to always consider the source of their information before accepting it as the truth. The fact that something good or bad is stated about a vitamin on the Internet, or even on the nightly news, necessarily does not make it true.

Recommended versus Therapeutic Dosage

Most of us have seen the Recommended Dietary Allowances (RDAs) on packaged food ingredient labels that were used for decades or the newer Recommended Daily Intakes (RDI). The RDI is used to determine the Daily Value (DV) of foods, which is printed on nutrition-facts labels in the United States and Canada and is regulated by the FDA and Health Canada, respectively.

Nutritionally minded doctors and nutritionists consider these RDAs, and now RDIs, inadequate. Why? Because these aren't based on what people need to be healthy, only what is needed to prevent obvious deficiencies. For example, the RDI for vitamin C of 60 milligrams per day is simply the amount needed to prevent scurvy, a disease that can happen when someone is profoundly vitamin C deficient for a long period of time. That's a pretty low bar! Nutritionally savvy practitioners suggest people consume 1,000 milligrams of vitamin C daily to be healthy. To treat a cold, I often recommend anywhere from 3,000 to 10,000 milligrams per day. The low levels of typical RDIs are not sufficient to promote *wellness.* When I recommend these higher levels of vitamin C, some patients respond, "I'll just drink lots of orange juice, Doc." I tell them that they had better ask Tropicana to deliver a tanker truck of orange juice with a very big straw to supply the vitamin C they will need to consume during the next week.

It's vital to grasp the distinction between using nutrients preventatively versus therapeutically. On this plan, you will be using supplements at appropriate *therapeutic* levels—to help you recover from an illness. When supplements are used to prevent an illness, the recommended levels are lower than when you have an active illness that must be treated.

For a more in-depth account of the therapeutic use of vitamins, nutrients, and herbs consider *The Encyclopedia of Natural Medicine* by Michael T. Murray, ND, and Joseph Pizzorno, ND, and *Prescriptions for Nutritional Healing* by Phyllis A. Balch, CNC. While there are more comprehensive and technical books available on this subject, they are often written for physicians. These books were written so that the average person can make sense of them.

Now that you better understand why vitamins and supplements are a crucial part of your healing, let's turn back to how you can use them to treat classic fibromyalgia and, in particular, how you can use them to boost your serotonin levels.

Using Supplements to Boost Serotonin

One reason that antidepressants help FM sufferers is that they enhance the effects of serotonin. (They can act via some of the same mechanisms as certain supplements—something doctors learned inadvertently.) The downside of this approach to raising serotonin levels, however, is that most pharmaceutical antidepressants have undesirable side effects. The newer classes of antidepressant drugs, like SSRIs (selective serotonin reuptake inhibitors) and SNRIs (serotonin and norepinephrine reuptake inhibitors), can also increase serotonin levels with fewer side effects than the older types—but they still have side effects, and not everyone responds to them in the same way.

I prefer to use what is known as precursor therapy, often along with other supports and medications, to boost serotonin. Precursor therapy means that instead of introducing a particular chemical that you want more of into the body, you introduce one of its building blocks instead. That way, the body can build the desired chemical, in this case, serotonin, on its own. A precursor to serotonin is 5-hydroxytryptophan (5-HTP). Available without a prescription, 5-HTP improves sleep and mood and reduces pain by raising serotonin levels;[7] 5-HTP should be taken with vitamin B_6 (preferably its active form, pyridoxal-5-phosphate) to support conversion to serotonin. The side effects—gastrointestinal cramping, nausea, and vivid dreams—are rare and manageable.

Mood Support Protocol

Follow these recommendations to boost serotonin and address many of the common FM symptoms we've discussed. You can take the following on a daily basis.

- 5-HTP, 50 to 100 milligrams per day with meals, increasing up to 300 milligrams as needed in divided dosages

- St. John's wort with 0.3 percent hypericin content, 300 milligrams three times a day (This is a botanical alternative to 5-HTP, and I normally do not use both together and generally avoid it if the patient is on other medications to prevent some reactions this herb may have with the clearance of some drugs.)

- SAMe (S-adenosylmethionine), 1,600 milligrams per day, to support the production of serotonin, norepinephrine, and dopamine (I use this occasionally, but not routinely with FM patients.)

- Melatonin, 3 to 9 milligrams 1 hour before bed to promote sleep; raise the dose over time as needed to achieve quality sleep (I often use a sustained-release version of melatonin to keep you asleep longer and help you cycle through all stages of sleep.)

- Phosphatidylserine, 50 to 100 milligrams per day, to promote calming neurotransmission (Phosphatidylcholine, inositol and choline, or glycerophosphocholine can all be used for the same purpose.)

- L-theanine, 100 to 200 milligrams per day (Though not commonly present in foods, this amino acid is found in herbal teas and green tea. It aids in the production of the calming neurotransmitter gamma-aminobutyric acid, or GABA, resulting in relaxation without overt sedation. It also lowers the physiological response to stress while improving attention.)

- Calming botanicals such as *Valeriana* (valerian), 100 to 200 milligrams per day; *Passiflora* (passion flower), 100 to 200 milligrams per day; *Scutellaria* (skullcap), 100 to 200 milligrams per day; and/or *Melissa* (lemon balm), 100 to 200 milligrams per day

When taking any herbal supplement, it's always best to consult with your health-care practitioner about possible herb-drug interactions. Caution should be used, for example, when taking 5-HTP in combination with SSRIs, SNRIs, or tramadol, as long-term combined use may lead to additional imbalances in the neurotransmitters. However, it's generally very safe to do so at typical doses of both the medication and 5-HTP, and I often use them in combination with great success while monitoring the person with lab testing and clinical observation.

Calming GABA Protocol

Another neurotransmitter that plays an important role in classic fibromyalgia is gamma-aminobutyric acid. GABA is an *inhibitory* neurotransmitter. That is, it has an inhibitory effect on the firing of neurons and supports a calm mood. GABA is synthesized from the amino acid glutamic acid. The prescription drugs alprazolam (Xanax) and clonazepam (Klonopin) increase the GABA effect in the nervous system.

To boost the functioning and levels of GABA, reduce anxiety and muscle tension, and improve sleep quality, follow this protocol.

- GABA, 100 to 200 milligrams two to three times per day (The fermented form of GABA, known as pharma-GABA, may work better than other forms to calm neurotransmission.)

- L-theanine, 100 to 200 milligrams per day

- Calming botanicals such as *Valeriana* (valerian), 100 to 200 milligrams per day; *Passiflora* (passion flower), 100 to 200 milligrams per day; *Scutellaria* (skullcap), 100 to 200 milligrams per day, and/or *Melissa* (lemon balm), 100 to 200 milligrams per day

Margaret's Story

Margaret was diagnosed with FM by a rheumatologist and put on Cymbalta, a SNRI used for treating depression, anxiety, and pain associated with diabetic peripheral neuropathy or fibromyalgia. In certain cases, this class of medications can be helpful, while other people with FM see little or no benefit. Side effects include nausea, dry mouth, constipation, loss of appetite, tiredness, drowsiness, or increased sweating. On Cymbalta, Margaret said she felt like a zombie, experiencing worse brain fog and memory lapses than prior to taking the medication. Plus, she was still depressed. I decided to add some 5-HTP, a form of the amino acid L-tryptophan, which helps the body produce more serotonin. Adding this simple supplement, at the correct dose, allowed the antidepressant to further enhance the effects of the higher levels of serotonin that were now being produced.

Margaret was also given a naturally fermented form of the neurotransmitter chemical GABA in a quick-acting chewable lozenge, helping to control her anxiety and allowing her to slowly taper off of Klonopin, an antianxiety medication she was also taking. By making these adjustments to her medications; adding some additional neurotransmitter support; putting her on a 21-day detoxification, anti-inflammatory, and antiallergenic diet; and giving her some other basic metabolic nutritional support, Margaret rapidly improved and reduced her body achiness, fatigue, brain fog, anxiety, and depression.

Adrenal Support

The level of hormones produced by the endocrine glands fluctuate with physical and emotional stress. In FM, the release of adrenal chemicals known as catecholamines, which are involved in the fight-or-flight response, is altered. This contributes to a state of constant—and exhausting—hypervigilance. Levels of cortisol (also involved in fight or flight and another chemical produced by the adrenals) are similarly affected. In classic FM, the release of cortisol is typically blunted in the morning, while levels are excessive late at night, which disrupts sleep.

When adding a natural adrenal support, it's important to conduct a simple urine test to see if catecholamines are high or low. These urine tests, known as organic acids tests, include vanilmandelate and homo-vanillate, both metabolites spilled into the urine due to the breakdown of catecholamines. Testing information is given on page 174.

The catecholamines include the neurotransmitters dopamine, epinephrine, and norepinephrine. These fluctuate with physical and emotional stress. If levels are high, I recommend that you use the following calming botanicals and nutrients.

- GABAergic and adaptogenic botanicals—herbs that act on GABA and the adrenal glands:

  Ashwagandha with 1.5 percent anolides, 100 to 200 milligrams per day

  Valeriana (valerian), 100 to 200 milligrams per day

  Passiflora (passion flower), 100 to 200 milligrams per day

  Melissa (lemon balm), 100 to 200 milligrams per day

- Phosphatidylserine, 100 to 200 milligrams per day

- L-theanine, 100 to 200 milligrams per day

If, on the other hand, a urine test shows catecholamines to be low, then stimulating rather than calming herbs and nutrients may be called for.

- Eleuthero with 0.8 percent eleutherosides, 200 milligrams per day*

- Korean or Chinese ginseng (*Panax ginseng*) with 5 percent ginsenosides, 100 to 200 milligrams per day*

- Golden root (*Rhodiola*) with 3 percent rosavins and 1 percent salidrosides, 100 to 200 milligrams per day

- Glycyrrhizin (licorice), 20 to 100 milligrams per day*

- Tyrosine (the N-acetyl tyrosine form preferred), 200 milligrams per day*

To conveniently order supplements for classic FM, check out the Fibro-Fix Classic FM packets and the individual products such as Sero-Tone, Neuro-Fix, and FibroMag available at FibroFix.com.

An Overview of Medications for Fibromyalgia

Treating all of the symptoms of central sensitization is the key focus of the three FDA-approved medications for FM pain: pregabalin (Lyrica), milnacipran (Savella), and duloxetine hydrochloride (Cymbalta). These medications may help some people with global widespread pain, indicative of classic fibromyalgia, but usually will not help those individuals inappropriately labeled as having FM.[8]

In 2007, pregabalin, an alpha-2-delta ($\alpha 2\delta$) ligand medication, originally used as an antiepileptic, became the first medication to gain FDA approval for the treatment of FM pain. Although, as with each of the three approved FM medications, it is not yet clear exactly how pregabalin works to relieve pain. It's currently believed to function by reducing nervous system hyperexcitability. Pain reduction may also result from decreased release of pro-pain neurotransmitters in the spinal cord and by modulating pain transmission in the spinal cord.

The other two medications approved for FM pain, duloxetine and milnacipran, are SNRIs originally developed as antidepressants. They are thought to amplify the ability of the neurotransmitters serotonin and norepinephrine to modulate pain-blocking pathways in the brain and spinal cord. Neither of these medications has been tested head-to-head (or against pregabalin, for that matter), which makes it difficult to assess relative effectiveness.

---

*Use tyrosine and stimulating adaptogenic botanicals—such as *Panax ginseng*, eleuthero, and licorice—with caution and only when low levels of the catecholamines have been confirmed in lab testing as they may worsen anxiety or insomnia.

OTHER MEDICATIONS FOR FM

There are other less commonly used medications for FM to address depression, pain, and other symptoms. Though not FDA-approved specifically for this purpose, they are nevertheless used by some physicians for the treatment of FM when people don't respond to the approved medications. These include:

- **Amitriptyline** (Elavil), known as a tricyclic antidepressant, is used for major depressive disorder as well as neuropathic pain disorders, fibromyalgia, irritable bowel syndrome, and migraines. It is rarely used as a first-line antidepressant nowadays, and while it used to be the most frequently used medication for FM patients, it has largely been replaced by newer medications. That is because it is highly toxic in overdose and is generally not tolerated as well as newer antidepressants, such as the SSRIs (selective serotonin reuptake inhibitors) and SNRIs (serotonin and norepinephrine reuptake inhibitors).

- **Nortriptyline** (Pamelor), also a tricyclic antidepressant, is used for the treatment of major depression. It is also used for the treatment of panic disorder, irritable bowel syndrome, neuropathic pain, migraines, chronic pain, and temporomandibular joint disorder. It can also aid in quitting smoking and in reducing the symptoms of ADHD. The most common side effects include dry mouth, sedation, constipation, increased appetite, mild blurred vision, tinnitus, euphoria, and mania. An occasional side effect is a rapid or irregular heartbeat. Alcohol may exacerbate some of its side effects and should be avoided. However, the incidence of side effects with nortriptyline is lower than with imipramine and amitriptyline, other drugs in the same class.

- **Trazodone** (Oleptro), a tetracyclic antidepressant, is used for major depression, with relatively mild side effects, and was originally welcomed as a treatment for geriatric patients with

(continued)

depression when it first became available. However, a side effect of trazodone, orthostatic hypotension (low blood pressure when getting up or sitting down), which may cause dizziness and increase the risk of falling, can have serious consequences for elderly patients. Trazodone has also been reported to have antianxiety properties. Many clinicians use low-dose trazodone as an alternative to benzodiazepines for the treatment of insomnia. Mania has been observed in association with trazodone treatment, including in patients with bipolar disorder and those with previous diagnoses of major depression.

☐ **Fluoxetine** (also known by the trade names Prozac and Sarafem, among others) is in the SSRI class. It is used for the treatment of major depressive disorder (including pediatric depression), obsessive-compulsive disorder (in both adults and children), and panic disorder. Side effects include abnormal dreams, lack of appetite, anxiety, diarrhea, dry mouth, GERD (gastroesophageal reflux disease), flulike symptoms, impotence, insomnia, decreased libido, nausea, nervousness, pharyngitis, rash, sinusitis, somnolence, sweating, tremor, vasodilatation, and yawning. Fluoxetine is considered the most stimulating of the SSRIs (that is, it is more likely to cause insomnia and agitation than the other SSRIs). It also appears to produce dermatologic reactions—such as urticaria (hives), rash, and itchiness—more often.

☐ **Sertraline** (Zoloft), also an SSRI, is used for major depression, obsessive-compulsive disorder, post-traumatic stress disorder, panic disorder, and social anxiety disorder. In studies, sertraline has fewer adverse effects than amitriptyline, nortriptyline, and imipramine, with the exception of nausea, which occurred more frequently. It also is associated with a higher rate of psychiatric side effects and diarrhea and tends to be more activating (that is, associated with a higher rate of anxiety, agitation, insomnia, etc.) than other SSRIs.

☐ **Low-dose naltrexone** (ReVia, Vivitrol) is an endorphin used to treat narcotic and opioid addiction. A recent Stanford University study using very low doses of naltrexone demonstrated a 30 percent reduction in pain for all 10 of the patients in this small study.[9] It is theorized that the positive outcomes observed in FM patients with low-dose naltrexone may be due not to its known ability to block opioid receptors but instead to its ability to alter immune-activating cells and lower inflammation of the microglia in the brain. It appears that while FM is not a disorder that causes widespread inflammation throughout the body, new evidence suggests that there may be small levels of inflammation deep within the brain. In effect, this may be a mechanism for addressing deep-brain pain, and low-dose naltrexone may be altering the pain in FM patients through this mechanism. Further investigation is called for, especially given the low cost and minimal side effects.

It is important to note that while these medications do benefit many classic fibromyalgia sufferers, a large percentage of classic FM patients will not see significant lessening of their pain. For these patients, other avenues clearly need to be explored, including other prescription medications and the nonprescription supplements and modalities discussed in this chapter. These approaches can very often effectively treat the underlying problems rather than simply masking pain.

Depression: Beyond Serotonin

As you have learned so far, depression, anxiety, and mood disorders are extremely common in FM, and serotonin plays a crucial role. However, an emerging body of scientific evidence clearly demonstrates that depression, anxiety, mood disorders, and global pain involve more than simply a deficiency of serotonin, GABA, or other neurotransmitters. Brain inflammation is another underlying factor.[10] Dietary changes, supplements, botanicals, lifestyle modifications, optimization of the GI flora, alleviation of leaky-gut syndrome, and medication have all been effective in lessening brain inflammation and improving the clinical outcomes of these disorders. Even though FM is not itself an overtly inflammatory disorder, new research suggests that FM and various mood disorders likely have common causes, including alterations in serotonin and other brain chemicals, micro-inflammation of the brain, and a history of stress, trauma, or abuse. And interesting correlations demonstrating this connection between stress, trauma, inflammation, depression, and FM continue to emerge.[11]

Even temporary stress can induce inflammation; studies show that students undergoing stressful examinations had higher levels of inflammation and cortisol as compared to when they were not under stress.[12] And public speaking has been shown to increase the inflammatory chemical known as IL-6 in presenters. Even troubled personal relationships can increase inflammation in partners.[13] Slowly, we are starting to understand how stress links to inflammation and how that, in turn, can contribute over time to the development of mood disorders, such as depression and anxiety, and ultimately to even more complex disorders, such as IBS and FM.[14]

Exercise and Relaxation

You are already reaping the benefits of gentle movement as part of the Fibro-Fix Foundational Plan. As I've noted, even movement as simple and relaxing as walking can improve pain levels, mood, and sleep. I recommend that you use a pedometer, with the ultimate goal of 10,000 steps each day. But it's important to respect your current limitations, and for some FM patients, 3 to 5 minutes of walking may be all that is possible at first. If you notice that you are getting short of breath to the point that you cannot hold a conversation with someone who is doing the activity with you, then you are exercising too vigorously for someone with classic FM.

I strongly encourage you to try any of the following forms of gentle movement, relaxation, and or stress reduction.

- Counseling
- Desensitization techniques
- Forgiveness therapy
- Guided imagery
- Heart-rate variability training
- Meditation
- Progressive muscle relaxation
- Tai chi or qigong
- Yoga

Please revisit the exercise program in Chapter 2 for detailed exercise plans. In particular, the mind-body exercises, such as progressive muscle relaxation, will be very helpful for you.

One of the pitfalls of beginning any exercise program if you have classic FM is that you may be out of shape due to pain, immobility, and low energy. As a result, you may be more prone to injury and fatigue. So starting slow and "leaving something in the tank" is essential. Going beyond your limit can also result in what is called postexertional fatigue—which can leave some people exhausted, in pain, and bedridden for several days. So no heroics, please. Nevertheless, if you have classic FM, a daily practice of centering and stress mitigation (which includes mild exercise) is a really important part of your program.

Putting It All Together

Let's take a look at what happens when you follow my total program for classic fibromyalgia.

Jennifer's Story

Jennifer, a 43-year-old real estate agent and mother of three, came to see me complaining of achiness, fatigue, and chronic constipation. She had pain globally rather than locally and no joint pain.

Jennifer had a history of anxiety and mild depression and a rough childhood. Her father was verbally abusive and loud and left the family after divorcing her mother when she was 12. Jennifer suspects that her father physically abused her mother while they were married. After he remarried and started a new family, he had little to do with her or her mother. Jennifer herself had several abusive boyfriends before getting married. Her husband was generally unsupportive and thought her condition was "all in her mind."

I gave her a physical exam, and she reported pain responses to digital pressure in all major muscle groups in all areas of her body—upper, lower, left, right, central, and peripheral. There was no joint swelling or pain. The results of an orthopedic and neurologic examination were normal.

Her vital signs, heart, lungs, and thyroid all appeared to be normal, and her muscles were generally not stiff, tight, or in spasm. There were a couple of myofascial trigger points in the upper shoulder/trapezius muscles, probably due to stress.

Her lab tests—including blood chemistry, complete blood count, thyroid panel, iron, and ferritin—were all normal, and markers for systemic inflammation and autoimmune disease were all negative.

In the absence of any other cause for her global pain, and with several clear indicators of fibromyalgia (including a past history of trauma, sleeplessness, anxiety, depression, and IBS), I determined that Jennifer had classic FM. Her course of treatment included: the 21-day Fibro-Fix Foundational Plan, including the detoxification program and anti-inflammatory and nonallergenic fresh food diet:

- ☐ 5-HTP (to increase serotonin levels for better mood, sleep, and lower pain perception)
- ☐ Melatonin (for improving sleep quality and lowering pain perception)
- ☐ GABA (to decrease anxiety, improve sleep, and lower pain perception)
- ☐ Calming, adrenal, and antianxiety herbals (for example, valerian, passion flower, ashwagandha, German chamomile)
- ☐ Calming nutrients (L-theanine, phosphatidylserine, magnesium)
- ☐ CoQ10 (for energy and mitochondrial metabolism support)
- ☐ Constipation support (magnesium citrate and fiber powder in morning)
- ☐ Mild range-of-motion and stretching exercises
- ☐ Daily meditation, guided imagery, and light yoga
- ☐ Psychological counseling with a counselor familiar with FM and post-traumatic stress disorder

After 1 month, Jennifer showed a 50 percent improvement in all symptoms and a 5-pound weight loss. After 60 days, she showed a 75 percent improvement in all symptoms and a 10-pound weight loss. After 6 months, she was largely free of symptoms, with only occasional mild achiness and fatigue, virtually no anxiety or depression, and no constipation. She was sleeping well. Jennifer continued with the counselor, entered marriage therapy, and reduced her supplement dosing by 50 percent. She has continued with an anti-inflammatory, fresh-food diet with no gluten-containing grains and uses a protein-based detox shake most days for breakfast. She has kept up her daily yoga and meditation practice and has a far more positive outlook on life in general.

An Emerging Therapeutic Approach

Every brain is unique, with its own pattern of electrical frequencies for efficient functioning. Trauma, both physical and nonphysical, may lead to disturbances in brain activity, including imbalances of these frequencies and amplitudes. Specifically, traumas or threats can lead to activation of autonomic nervous system responses, including sympathetic (fight-or-flight) or parasympathetic (freeze or withdrawal) responses, which are designed to help you survive the event. If the brain circuitry involved with managing the responses remains chronically activated, the physiological changes that accompany this can contribute to an unhealthy pattern of hypervigilance and ultimately lead to the symptoms of illnesses like FM.

Brain-Feedback Technology

Lee Gerdes and Brain State Technologies have developed a noninvasive brain-feedback technology that facilitates relaxation and balances brain frequencies by using auditory tones.[15] The first step in the HIRREM (high-resolution, relational, resonance-based, electroencephalic mirroring) therapy process is to assess the brain's electrical pattern. This is done by making very brief recordings of the brainwaves at six or more locations on the scalp while the recipient is both at rest and carrying out a task. The assessment includes 1-minute recordings at each location with the eyes first closed, then partially open, and then fully open while performing a specific mental task (for example, recalling numbers or reading a passage). This provides a map of frequencies and amplitudes within the brain both at rest and while interacting with the environment, allowing for the identification of imbalances.

HIRREM protocols (that is, the auditory signal patterns) are different for each patient, with subsequent protocols based on initial responses, and are done with the recipient sitting or reclining in a comfortable chair. Sensors are placed on the scalp at specific locations, allowing the computer to observe the brainwaves and identify a dominant frequency at a particular moment. This frequency is assigned an auditory tone, which is played back via earbuds in nearly real-time (as little as 8 milliseconds). The brainwaves are constantly changing, so the recipient hears a series of tones. It appears that the brain quickly recognizes that the tones reflect what is going on in the brain at the time. By giving the brain a chance to listen to itself via this acoustic stimulation, it will, on its own, tend to self-optimize, usually resulting in an electrical shift toward improved balance and quieting. There is no cognitive activity required by the recipient, no requirement to relive a traumatic event, and no attempt to force the brain into a specific pattern.

Although the number of sessions varies, most individuals receive at least 10. While more research is needed to assess the long-term outcomes of this therapy, the results are promising so far, with many patients reporting a decrease in pain and anxiety as well as improved sleep. For more about HIRREM and ongoing research trials on this therapy, visit wakehealth.edu/research/neurology/HIRREM/about/about-HIRREM.htm. Many other similar technologies using biofeedback methods to retrain brain responses and wave patterns are also being used by integrative and functional medicine physicians specializing in stress and pain-related disorders.

Conclusion

Please remember that my program of dietary and lifestyle changes, nutritional supplements, and nutriceuticals addresses the issues most commonly seen in classic fibromyalgia. People with chronic pain and fatigue should always be screened and treated in the event that other diseases (for example, anemia, hypothyroid, or autoimmune disease), functional/metabolic disorders (such as mitochondrial dysfunction or nutritional deficiencies), or musculoskeletal problems are present. It is very common for muscle and joint as well as metabolic problems to compound FM. Please read the next three chapters for more information about these categories, or buckets, so you and your health-care practitioner can develop your customized program for a life that is pain-free and full of vitality.

CHAPTER 5

THE STRUCTURAL FIX

Even doctors are fooled by the variety of illnesses that masquerade as classic fibromyalgia. In Chapter 3, we looked at three kinds of disorders that mimic FM—musculoskeletal, functional, and conventional diseases. You then filled out a questionnaire to determine if your condition is likely classic fibromyalgia or something else. In Chapter 4, we looked at classic fibromyalgia and my approach to treating it. If the results of the questionnaire showed that you do *not* have classic fibromyalgia, I recommend that you read this and the next two chapters carefully. In particular, if you think your issue is muscular or structural, pay close attention to the information and protocols in this chapter. With a better understanding of this very different kind of pain syndrome, you will learn how to become pain-free.

When several unique muscles and joints each produce pain, it's natural in certain cases to assume that they are all connected in one body-wide pain condition. This assumption leads many people (and their doctors) to believe that they suffer from classic FM. But in my experience, quite often they don't. It's a little like a school classroom where there are a few bad apples. Out of frustration, the teacher doesn't notice the individual troublemakers anymore. She just looks out over the class and sees nothing but trouble! Misdiagnosing the problem, she makes them *all* stay after school.

It is common for doctors to misdiagnose musculoskeletal conditions. In a study I mentioned earlier, of the 252 people referred to a clinic for global pain treatment, over one-third of those had a musculoskeletal condition, not classic FM.[1] This misdiagnosis frequently occurs with seniors. The normal aches and pains of aging, along with muscle and joint problems and arthritis, are often misdiagnosed as fibromyalgia.[2]

From my work with thousands of people, I've found that a musculoskeletal issue can cause a wide range of symptoms, which can usually be resolved by the program in this chapter. The program includes the diet, supplement protocols, gentle movement and exercise, and relaxation practices you are already following on the Fibro-Fix Foundation Plan. In this chapter, you will learn why and when to add treatment by a physical therapist, chiropractor, acupuncturist, and/or massage therapist and how at-home therapies can also be used. The right combination of therapies can ease or eliminate musculoskeletal problems entirely. Although this pathway to healing is not usually suggested by conventional doctors, you will learn all you need to know to pursue my approach here.

Two years ago, Leon injured his lower back in a work-related accident. Compounding that, he had whiplash from a previous car accident. Then in another unrelated incident, he twisted one of his knees while walking down the stairs. Leon went to the chiropractor for the back injury and received massage for the whiplash. But after the knee injury, his girlfriend insisted he go see her primary care physician.

When the doctor asked, "Where do you hurt?" Leon answered, "I seem to hurt everywhere . . . my lower back, my neck, my knee . . ." But because he perceived his pain as widespread, Leon did not think to trace it back to those separate injuries. Even though he was too distracted, or in too much pain, to understand those connections, his doctor should have probed more deeply and found out about the previous accidents. But the busy doctor did not take the time (or have the right training) to sort through these three separate and distinct muscle and joint issues. Accepting the response from Leon that he "hurt all over," while never confirming this with a hands-on exam, she diagnosed him with FM and prescribed an antidepressant and a pain medication—as is commonly done. The result was that the pain lessened but did not disappear, and the cause (in this case, the multiple causes) of Leon's supposed "widespread pain" remained undetected.

Types of Musculoskeletal Pain

About 20 to 30 percent of people who have what they perceive to be a global pain issue actually have a condition caused by musculoskeletal misalignments and injuries or by myofascial pain syndrome.

Typically, the types of musculoskeletal pain that mimic FM arise from:

- Misalignments and injuries of the muscles, bones, and joints
- Muscle knots (trigger points)
- Disc degeneration
- Nerve root irritation or compression (pinched nerves)
- Postural distortions
- Toxic load
- Tendonitis/tendonosis

Let's take a look at these conditions one by one.

Misalignments and Injuries of the Muscles, Bones, and Joints

Pain and misalignment can arise from poor posture or the stresses and activities of daily life, such as sitting at a computer all day, driving, or lifting something incorrectly. In Leon's case, it came from a series of injuries that had a synergistic effect.

Trigger Points

In Chapter 3, I explained the difference between tender points and trigger points. You may recall that tender points, often used to diagnose fibromyalgia, are not caused by inflammation or injury to the musculoskeletal system. They originate from the central nervous system.

HOW DO TENDER POINTS FEEL?

Tender points definitely hurt; when someone presses them with a finger, you will flinch or pull back. But the root cause is not in that area of the body. Think of it this way: If your flight to Chicago is cancelled, it may be because there is a problem with your aircraft, or it may be because a giant weather system has shut down all the air traffic in the Midwest. If you've got classic FM, you're dealing with the giant weather system, not the local equipment.

Tender points, as I have pointed out, should not be confused with trigger points. So if your doctor or practitioner starts referring to the "trigger points" activated by fibromyalgia, he is basically under- or misinformed, and you should get a second opinion.

Unlike tender points, trigger points really are linked to a musculoskeletal condition. They are often a symptom of myofascial pain syndrome—a disorder involving the fascia, muscles, and soft tissue.

HOW DO TRIGGER POINTS FEEL?

Trigger points are the lumps, knots, or tight bands you sometimes find in your muscles after you have been bruised or injured or have overexercised. You may also develop them if you've just had too much stress. Trigger points can also come from poor posture. For example, if you spend your days at a stressful job hunched over a computer and drive to that job in traffic for over an hour each way, it would not be surprising if you developed trigger points—especially in the neck and upper shoulders. The pain from trigger points, you may remember, can radiate out—or in doctor-speak, be "referred"—from the main site of the knot in the muscle. And when there are several areas of referred pain overlapping, you've got something that seems global—but isn't.

Trigger points can be treated with various forms of hands-on physical medicine, such as deep pressure massage, physical therapy, chiropractic, and acupuncture. I will discuss these modalities later on in this chapter. In contrast, the tender points found with classic FM won't respond to manual massage or therapies because they are not muscle problems. Many people keep going for more body work and physical treatments when they actually have the tender points of classic FM, enduring the pain of the therapy without any real chance of its improving their condition. In reality, it's a form of minor torture without any lasting benefit. They need an entirely different approach, which I discussed in the preceding chapter.

Disc Degeneration

Degeneration of one or more of the spinal discs can cause acute or chronic back pain. The spinal discs consist of cartilage that separates the vertebrae of the spine, act as shock absorbers between the vertebrae, and allow the spine some flexibility. The pain from a degenerated disc sometimes radiates to the arms, hips, buttocks, and thighs, depending on its location in the spine. There may also be sporadic tingling or weakness through the legs, knees, hands, and fingers. Chronic neck pain can also originate from the spine and radiate to the head, shoulders, arms, and hands.

Degenerative disc disease can often be successfully treated without surgery. Physical therapy, chiropractic and osteopathic treatments, anti-inflammatory medications, and, in more serious cases, traction or spinal injections can usually provide adequate relief.

There are also new treatments emerging, including glucosamine injections, artificial disc replacement, and adult stem-cell therapies.

Pinched Nerves

A pinched nerve occurs when surrounding tissues—such as bones, cartilage (discs), muscles, or tendons—apply too much pressure to a nerve. This pressure disrupts the nerve's function. Signs and symptoms of a pinched nerve include:

- Numbness or decreased sensation
- Sharp, aching, or burning pain, sometimes radiating outward
- Paresthesia (a "pins and needles" sensation)
- Muscle weakness
- Loss of normal deep-tendon reflexes (assessed with a reflex hammer by a doctor)

Pinched nerves can occur at many sites in your body. A herniated disc in your lower spine, for example, can put pressure on a lumbar nerve root, causing pain that radiates down the back of your leg. A pinched nerve in your neck can cause pressure down your arm. Pressure on a nerve in your wrist can lead to carpal tunnel syndrome, pain, and numbness in your hand and fingers.

With rest and other conservative treatments, most people recover from a pinched nerve within a few days or weeks. In certain cases, surgery may be needed.

Postural Distortions

Our bodies are complex structural mechanical systems, and imbalances in one area produce compensations—also imbalanced—in other regions. Postural deviations can stress the body and cause pain in a number of ways. A postural distortion can be:

- **Primary:** The distortion occurs in the same region of the body in which the pain is experienced. An example of this is someone developing chronic neck pain from constantly slouching and not sitting or standing up with good posture.

- **Secondary:** This is caused by a postural distortion elsewhere in the body. For example, any postural distortion of the pelvis will immediately bring about a compensatory distortion of the spine, which may result in mid-back or even neck pain. The distortion could be from an old knee or ankle injury that is causing you to walk differently, putting excessive stress on your hip and pelvis, ultimately resulting in severe chronic hip pain.

Postural distortion can also occur when the head is not balanced over the shoulders and therefore not protected from the downward pull of gravity. When that happens, your head becomes a 6-pound weight that forces the muscles of the neck to contract just to hold it up, resulting in daily neck and upper-shoulder pain.

A torsion, or twist, in the pelvis can lead to a postural distortion, as well. The torsion can result in differences in functional leg length, causing the body to lean to one side and the muscles in the waist and lower back to contract, ultimately leading to low-back pain.

Toxic Load

Most people don't realize that the toxins held in the bodily tissues, fat, bloodstream, and cells can also cause muscle pain. Just as excess lactic acid in your cells causes the aches and pains you feel after overexerting yourself in exercise, toxins present in the food we eat and the products we use (not to mention those released by industrial activities) can also burden our bodies and cause muscle pain. The Fibro-Fix Foundational Plan is designed to lower your toxic load. In Chapter 8, I discuss how to adopt a lifestyle that keeps your body as free of toxins as possible.

Tendonitis

Tendonitis is inflammation of the tendons. Tendons are the cordlike tissues that connect muscle to bone. Tendonitis is common in sports, among both professionals and weekend athletes. For example, rock climbers get it in their fingers or elbows, swimmers in their shoulders, runners and jumpers in their Achilles tendon, basketball and volleyball players in their patellar tendon (the tendon that connects the kneecap to the shinbone).

Tendonitis can produce aches, pains, joint stiffness, and even a burning sensation around the inflamed tendon. There may also be swelling, heat, and redness.

Tendon injuries are commonly treated with nonsteroidal anti-inflammatory drugs (NSAIDs), like ibuprofen, and rest. Compression is sometimes recommended. Depending on where the injury is, ice and elevation may be appropriate and effective. Physical and occupational therapy and sometimes orthotics and braces can be helpful. While recovery is usually pretty quick—anywhere from a few days to a few months for more serious cases—if tendonitis is not completely healed, it can turn into a chronic condition called tendinosis. Prolotherapy and platelet-rich plasma injections are often used with good results in tendinosis.

Platelet-rich plasma (PRP) injections are a specially prepared mixture of your own blood platelets (platelets are the cells in your blood that cause clotting); your blood plasma, the liquid part of your blood; and anesthetic. PRP injections work by providing the injured or inflamed area with a richer supply of your own blood, and its natural healing factors, thereby stimulating growth and repair.

Prolotherapy uses a similar, yet different, technique. It involves repeated injections of some irritating but harmless substance like dextrose into a joint space, weakened ligament, or tendon insertion. The injections cause inflammation, which in turn stimulates more rapid healing, along with thickening and strengthening of the ligament or tendon.

In the remainder of this chapter, I'll discuss some protocols you can follow yourself to help with musculoskeletal pain. By combining these protocols with the Fibro-Fix Foundational Plan and some hands-on body-centered therapies (such as chiropractic, acupuncture, massage, and physical therapy), you, like many of my patients, could feel better within a month. For some, symptoms can resolve in up to 3 months.

The Structural Fix Plan

If you have musculoskeletal pain, there is a lot you can do even before you know the specific cause of your condition. Start with the Fibro-Fix Foundational Plan, discussed in Chapter 2. This plan provides a basic foundation for healing by removing inflammatory and allergenic foods

IDENTIFYING THE SOURCE OF YOUR NECK OR SHOULDER PAIN

Neck pain: To find out if your neck pain comes from a musculoskeletal problem in the neck muscles or joints, gently turn your neck fully to the right and left. Next look up toward the ceiling and down toward the floor. If any of those movements triggers your pain, this suggests a structural problem. This chapter will guide you to the right kind of physical rehabilitation support for your pain.

Shoulder pain: To find out if your shoulder pain comes from a musculoskeletal problem in the shoulder muscles or joints, first gently and slowly raise your arm toward the ceiling. Next, try to reach back behind you to the center of your mid-back. If either of these movements causes the pain to worsen, this will confirm that the pain arises from a structural problem, such as a misalignment of (or injury to) your shoulder joint or problems with the rotator cuff muscles or tendons. Both of these can be alleviated by specific manual therapies or by natural or pharmaceutical anti-inflammatories. However, surgery is sometimes required. If there is no movement or position that makes your pain worse, it may not be coming from a muscle, tendon, or joint. Instead, there may be other sources of the pain.

along with chemicals from your diet. It will also nourish you with plenty of protein and vitamins needed for detoxification and healing. But beyond that, if your issue is musculoskeletal, follow my Structural Fix Plan, outlined below, which consists of:

- Stretching and mobility exercises

- Appropriate supplements

- Stress reduction techniques

- Professional support

Stretching and Mobility Exercises

This section is intended to get you back in touch with your body. You may be thinking that by living with chronic pain and fatigue, you are *constantly* in touch with your body, even if it's only to feel how restricted your movements are or how tender certain spots are. But this attitude can lead you to neglect one of the most powerful healing modalities for both body and mind—touch, and its most common form, massage. Your body may be so sensitive that the mere *thought* of a massage is painful. If that's the case, there's good news: Massage can be a form of self-care—that is, you can perform a massage on yourself, applying only as much or as little pressure as you are comfortable with.

THE BENEFITS OF USING A FOAM ROLLER

The easiest way to accomplish this is with a foam roller, a simple piece of equipment you can find at any sporting goods store or on many Internet sites. A foam roller is a lightweight cylinder typically made of Styrofoam or a similar material. You simply place it on the floor and roll various muscle groups along it, applying whatever amount of pressure feels appropriate. Foam rolling improves circulation and helps release muscle tightness that may be limiting your range of motion.

It may also be helpful for moving lymph through the body. Unlike blood, which moves through the blood vessels each time the heart beats, lymph has no dedicated pump. It only moves when you do. Lymph is propelled through the lymphatic vessels via muscle contractions and body movement. The stretching and mobility work you do will help, but this type of self-care tissue massage can take it even further, particularly if you are not able to walk or engage in other physical activity on a regular basis. Keeping lymph moving is important for preventing some forms of edema (swelling). And lymph is a key component of the immune system, transporting critical defense compounds throughout the body, so you don't want it pooling or stagnating.

The beauty of movement exercises that involve foam rolling or self-massage is that *you* control the pace and pressure. Even the best massage therapist can't get inside your head to experience sensations exactly as you do, because only *you* know exactly how a certain motion makes you feel and when your body could benefit from more or less of certain movements. Foam rolling—once only a kind of secret gem that professional athletes and physical therapists knew about—is now available to everyone.

You can find numerous free tutorials online demonstrating different ways to best use a foam roller. While I highly recommend you obtain a foam roller, if you do not want to purchase one you can improvise one at home (although much harder to use and not as effective) with a tightly rolled-up large towel, or simply run the muscle groups along the edge of a chair or couch.

Foam rolling and other forms of self-myofascial release can also help you identify possible sources of referred pain, which you might not have been aware of previously. Referred pain occurs when pressure applied to one area of the body is felt elsewhere, possibly even somewhere seemingly unrelated. (Of course, the two painful areas are related *internally*, through the network of nerves that extend throughout the body.) Identifying referred pain may help you realize that you have myofascial pain syndrome—a problem locally in the muscles, fascia, and soft tissues—and not a pain *perception* issue, which is at the heart of global pain syndromes like classic fibromyalgia.

GENERAL GUIDELINES FOR PROPER FOAM ROLLING

- Apply light to moderate pressure to a muscle or muscle group using your body weight against the roller.

- Roll at your own pace, but keep it slow. A good place to start is about an inch per second.

- When you come upon areas that are especially tight or painful, pause and maintain pressure on that site while you attempt to relax for several seconds. You will feel the tension slowly releasing.

- If you find spots that you can't apply pressure to directly because they are too painful, shift your position slightly and apply pressure instead to the surrounding tissue. Over time, the whole area will loosen up.

- Remember: There is a difference between pain and discomfort. According to natural-movement expert Jeff Kuhland, "think of it like the pain you get while stretching. It should be uncomfortable but not unbearable, and when you are done, it should feel better." Let your body guide you as to when and where the foam-rolling technique is helping, and when it is making you feel worse.

PROPER BREATHING

As we discussed in Chapter 2, proper breathing during exercise is important and enhances the outcome of the exercise. Diaphragmatic breathing is a recommended breathing technique to incorporate while exercising. When breathing this way, the stomach expands as you inhale through the nose (as opposed to the chest expanding) and the stomach deflates during exhalation through the mouth. This can be practiced by simply placing a hand on your stomach and feeling it inflate and deflate when taking a breath. Apply this breathing technique during all exercises.

MOVEMENT AND STRENGTHENING ROUTINE

The next pages are instructions for a gentle movement and strengthening routine, incorporating basic and inexpensive equipment, to help you alleviate your musculoskeletal pain.

Equipment Needed

- Exercise floor mat (optional)
- Foam roller
- Large exercise ball
- Small exercise ball (a tennis ball also works)
- Strap or belt

1. NECK RETRACTION AND SHOULDER PRESS

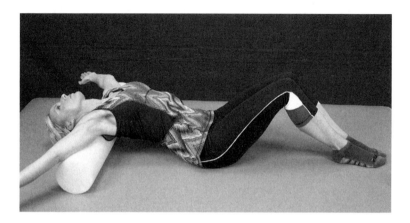

Targets: Neck, upper back, shoulders

Purpose: To reduce neck and shoulder pain; reduce muscle tightness; restore normal, healthy posture; and increase neck and shoulder mobility

Instructions: Lie on your back with a foam roller or rolled towel placed behind the base of your neck and your knees bent. Stretch your arms out horizontally, palms up. Gently press your head and shoulders in a backward direction (toward the exercise mat or floor). Hold this position for three diaphragmatic breaths. Repeat for a total of 10 repetitions.

2. NECK ROLL

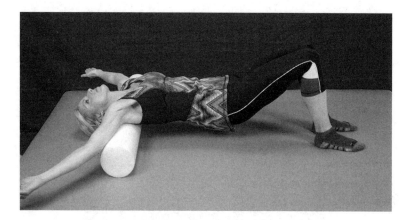

Targets: Neck, upper back, shoulders

Purpose: To reduce neck and shoulder pain; reduce muscle tightness; restore normal, healthy posture; and increase neck mobility

Instructions: While lying on your back, with knees bent and arms stretched out behind your head, place the foam roller behind the base of your neck and lift your head off the mat or floor. Starting from the base of your neck, slowly roll your upper body onto the foam roller in an upward direction until the foam roller is underneath your shoulder blades. Hold this position for 1 to 2 seconds, and then roll your upper body in a downward direction until the foam roller is underneath your neck. Throughout the exercise, maintain your head and neck in a slightly extended position. Continue this motion while engaged in diaphragmatic breathing for approximately 3 to 5 minutes. Adjust your exercise time based on your tolerance and comfort level.

3. SHOULDER-BLADE PRESS AND HEAD TILT

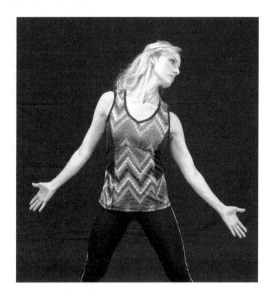

Targets: Head, neck, shoulders, upper back, mid-back

Purpose: To reduce neck and shoulder pain; reduce muscle tightness; improve mobility; and restore normal, healthy posture

Instructions: Stand with your legs shoulder width apart and your knees slightly bent, palms faced outward. Gently squeeze your shoulder blades together and tilt your head back at a 45-degree angle toward the right side (right ear toward right shoulder). Hold for three slow, deep breaths, inhaling through the nose and exhaling through the mouth. Return your head to a neutral (center) position. Next, squeeze your shoulder blades together and bring your head back in at a 45-degree angle toward the left side (left ear toward your left shoulder). Repeat the same breathing sequence. Bring your head to a neutral (central) position. This is 1 repetition. Repeat for a total of 10 repetitions.

4. DOOR-FRAME SHOULDER STRETCH

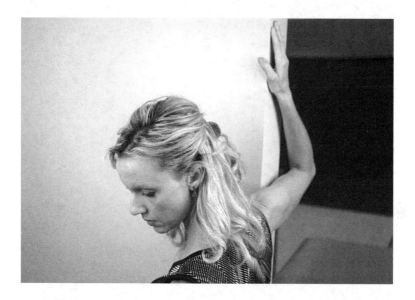

Targets: Shoulder, neck, chest

Purpose: To reduce pain; restore normal, healthy posture; improve mobility; and reduce muscle tightness

Instructions: Facing the doorway, stand on the right side of the door parallel to the door jam. Place your right arm on the jam with your hand slightly above your head and your elbow slightly bent. Take one small step forward with your left foot, and with your head upright, rotate your chin over your left shoulder. Hold this position for three diaphragmatic breaths. Return to the neutral (central) position, and repeat for a total of 10 repetitions. Face the opposite side and repeat the same sequence with your left arm on the door jam and your right foot forward.

5. SEATED BALL ROTATION

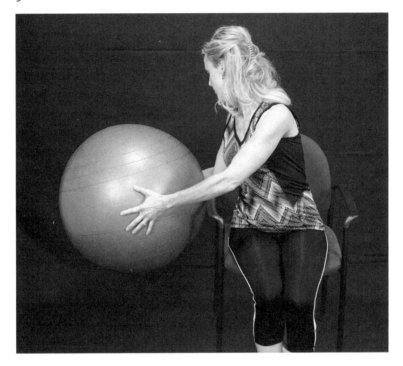

Targets: Neck, upper back, mid-back, shoulders

Purpose: To reduce pain and muscle tightness; restore normal, healthy posture; and improve mobility

Instructions: Seated in a chair, with your lower back in a slightly extended (arched backward) position and an exercise ball in your hand, rotate to your right side, positioning your hands and the ball just behind your right hip. With your head extended slightly backward, rotate your chin over your right shoulder. Hold this position for three diaphragmatic breaths. Return to the starting position. Repeat the same sequence on the left side. This is 1 repetition. Repeat for a total of 10 repetitions.

6. MID-BACK FORWARD FLEX

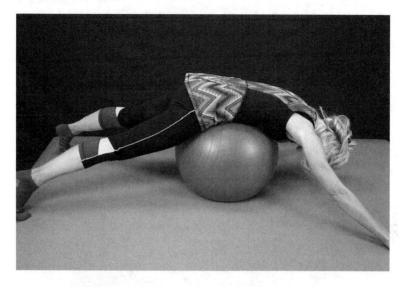

Targets: Mid-back, lower back

Purpose: To reduce mid- and low-back pain, improve mobility, and reduce muscle tightness

Instructions: Kneeling on the exercise mat, with your chest on the large exercise ball, roll forward until your arms and shoulder blades are extended over the ball. Hold this position for three diaphragmatic breaths. Return to the starting position. Repeat for a total of 10 repetitions.

7. MID-BACK SIDE BEND

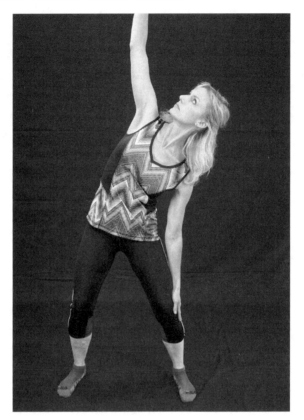

Targets: Mid-back, lower back, shoulders

Purpose: To reduce mid- and low-back pain; reduce muscle tightness; improve mobility; and restore healthy, normal posture

Instructions: In a standing position, with your legs shoulder-width apart, knees slightly bent, pelvis slightly rotated backward, and your arms at your sides, slide the fingers of your left hand down toward your left knee while bringing your right arm overhead and side-bending the upper body to the left. Your head and neck should be extended backward slightly and rotated upward to the right. Hold this position for three diaphragmatic breaths. Return to the starting position. Repeat the same sequence side-bending to the right. This is 1 repetition. Repeat for a total of 10 repetitions. (This exercise can also be performed sitting in a chair with ankles, knees, and hips bent at 90 degrees.)

8. LOW-BACK ROTATION WITH A BALL

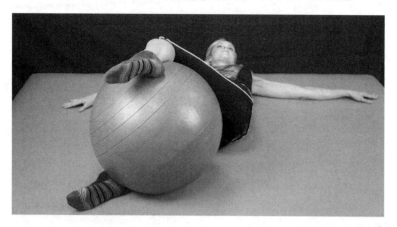

Targets: Lower back, mid-back, hips

Purpose: To reduce low-back and mid-back pain; improve mobility; reduce muscle tightness; and restore normal, healthy posture

Instructions: Lie on your back with a rolled towel placed behind the base of your neck, your arms spread out horizontally from your sides, the ball under your knees, and your knees aligned with your shoulders. (To hold the ball in place while doing this exercise, slightly squeeze in with both legs.) Rotate the ball to the right until you feel a minimal stretch (pull) in your low-back muscles. Hold this position for three diaphragmatic breaths. Return to the starting position. Repeat the same sequence on the left side. This is 1 repetition. Repeat for a total of 10 repetitions.

9. LOW-BACK ROLL

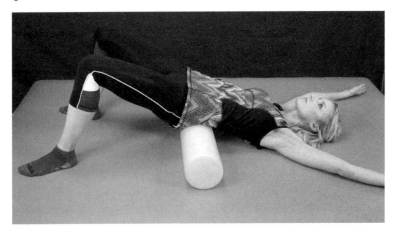

Targets: Lower back

Purpose: To reduce low-back pain; improve mobility; reduce muscle tightness; and restore normal, healthy posture

Instructions: Lie on your back with your knees bent. Place the foam roller under your lower back. Spread your arms outward above your head and place on the floor. Make sure to keep your lower back slightly arched during this exercise. Roll your body in a downward direction until the foam roller is under your mid-back. Hold this position for 1 to 2 seconds, followed by rolling your body in an upward direction until the foam roller is underneath your lower back. This exercise can be repeated while engaged in diaphragmatic breathing for 3 to 5 minutes. Adjust the exercise time based on your tolerance and comfort level.

10. HAMSTRING STRETCH

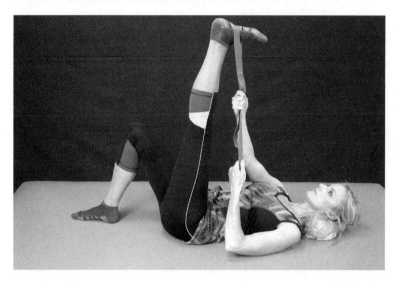

Targets: Hips, lower back

Purpose: To reduce hip and low-back pain, improve mobility, and reduce muscle tightness

Instructions: Lie on your back, with a rolled towel placed behind the base of your neck, your pelvis slightly rotated downward, your right knee bent, and your left leg straight. With a strap or belt around your left foot and your toes pointed toward your head, pull your left leg in an upward direction until you feel a minimal stretch (pulling) sensation in the left hamstring region. Hold this position for five diaphragmatic breaths. Bring your leg back onto the mat. Repeat for a total of 10 repetitions. Repeat the same sequence with your right leg.

11. HIP ROTATION

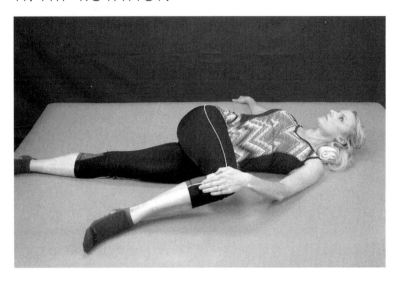

Targets: Hips, sides of upper thighs (iliotibial band), lower back, mid-back

Purpose: To reduce hip, low-back, and mid-back pain; improve mobility; and reduce muscle tightness

Instructions: Lying on your back with a rolled towel placed under the base of your neck, bring your right knee in an upward direction and with your left hand, gently rotate your right hip toward the left side of your body. Stop when you feel a minimal pulling/stretching sensation on the outside of your right hip and leg. Rotate your head and neck toward your right shoulder. Hold this position for three diaphragmatic breaths. Repeat the same sequence, rotating your left hip toward the right side of body. This is 1 repetition. Repeat for a total of 10 repetitions.

12. LATERAL HIP ROLL

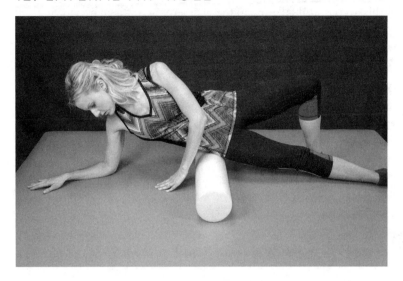

Targets: Hips, sides of upper thighs (iliotibial band)

Purpose: To reduce hip and lateral (outside) thigh pain, restore hip mobility, and reduce muscle tightness

Instructions: Lying on your right side, with a foam roller placed underneath your right hip, roll toward your right knee, holding for 1 to 2 seconds, followed by rolling back toward your hip. Continue this motion while engaged in diaphragmatic breathing for approximately 3 to 5 minutes. Increase or decrease the exercise time based on your tolerance and comfort level.

Treating Your Trigger Points

This section will take you to the next level of self-help by showing you how to treat some of the most common trigger points. There is no danger in doing this if you use your body's reaction as your guide. If it hurts too much, don't do it! Alter the pressure based on how your body feels. Start easy and work your way up to more pressure over time.

Equipment Needed

- Small, compressible ball (a tennis ball is perfect)
- Foam roller

1. NECK TRIGGER POINT EXERCISE

Targets: Upper trapezius muscles

Instructions: Standing with your back against a wall, place a small, compressible ball between your neck and the wall, positioning the ball at the location of the trigger point and taut muscle fibers. With your legs slightly bent and your neck pressed against the ball, roll your neck in an upward and downward (vertical) direction by slightly bending and straightening your knees. Then, shift your weight from side to side to roll your neck in a sideways (horizontal) direction. This will promote a rolling-type pressure on the trigger point and taut muscle fibers. Alternate rolling in vertical and horizontal directions for approximately 1.5 to 2 minutes.

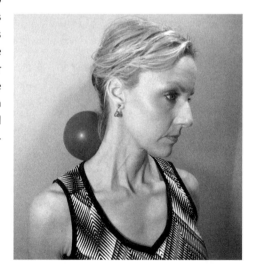

2. NECK AND UPPER-BACK TRIGGER POINT EXERCISE

Targets: Levator scapula muscle

Instructions: Standing with your back against a wall, place a small, compressible ball on the trigger point and taut muscle fibers located between the lower neck and scapula (wing bone). With your legs slightly bent and your neck/upper back pressed against the ball, roll your neck/upper back in an upward and downward (vertical) direction by slightly bending and straightening your knees. Then, shift your weight from side to side to roll your neck/upper back in a sideways (horizontal) direction. This will place pressure on the trigger point and taut muscle fibers. Alternate rolling in vertical and horizontal directions for approximately 1.5 to 2 minutes.

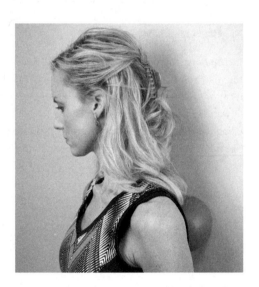

3. MID-BACK TRIGGER POINT EXERCISE

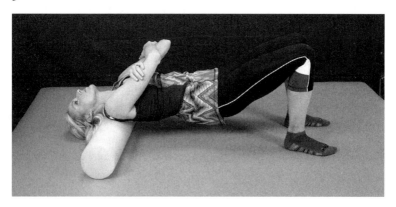

Targets: Erector spinae muscles

Instructions: Lie on your back with your knees bent, your pelvis elevated off the mat, and the foam roller placed underneath your mid-back region at the location of the trigger point and taut muscle fibers. Roll your mid-back in an upward and downward direction on the roller by slightly bending and straightening your knees. This will place pressure on the trigger point and taut muscle fibers. Continue foam rolling for approximately 1.5 to 2 minutes.

4. LOW-BACK TRIGGER POINT EXERCISE

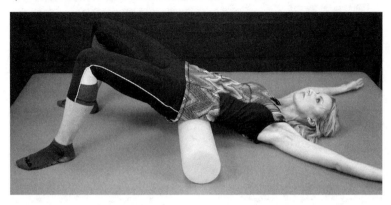

Targets: Musculo-aponeurosis of the lumbar spine

Instructions: Lie on your back with your knees bent and the foam roller placed underneath your lower back at the location of the trigger point and taut muscle fibers. Roll your lower back in an upward and downward direction on the roller by slightly bending and straightening your knees. Extend your arms outward and upward above your head. This exercise will place pressure on the trigger point and taut muscle fibers. Continue foam rolling for approximately 1.5 to 2 minutes.

5. BUTTOCKS TRIGGER POINT EXERCISE

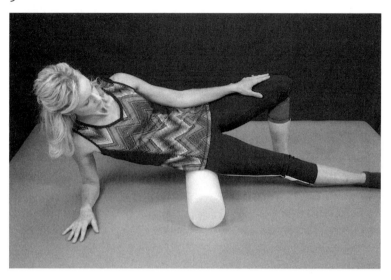

Targets: Gluteus medius and maximus, piriformis muscles

Instructions: If treating the right buttock, position your body midway between lying on your back and side-lying (at a 45-degree angle) on your right side. Place the foam roller under your right buttock at the location of the trigger point and taut muscle fibers. Your left leg will be bent, your right leg straight, and your right elbow bent with your body weight resting on the roller and elbow. Roll your buttock in an upward and downward direction on the roller by shifting your weight on your elbow and using your left foot and right forearm to slightly push and pull your body weight. This will place pressure on the trigger point and taut muscle fibers. Continue foam rolling for approximately 1.5 to 2 minutes. Repeat the same sequence for treating the left buttock.

6. CALF TRIGGER POINT EXERCISE

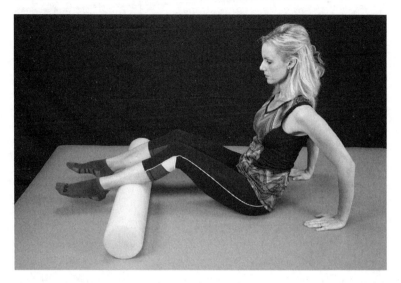

Targets: Gastrocnemius muscle

Instructions: If treating your right calf, sit on the floor with your arms extended behind your body and your right leg straight and your left leg bent. Place the roller under your right calf at the location of the trigger point and taut muscle fibers. Roll your right calf in an upward and downward direction on the roller by pushing with your left foot and extended arms. This will place pressure on the trigger point and taut muscle fibers. Continue foam rolling for approximately 1.5 to 2 minutes. Repeat the same sequence for treating the left calf. You may also choose to roll both legs at once as you become more proficient, as shown.

Appropriate Supplements

As I've discussed earlier, conventional Western medicine has always downplayed the importance of vitamins and other supplements and has instead invested its efforts and money in the drug model of health care. (If you haven't read this discussion, I suggest you read it now, starting on page 94.) You may have even heard that vitamins are a waste of money and all the nutrition you could ever need is in your food. Although this sounds like a logical premise, and may have been true once, it isn't anymore. For one thing, because of depleted soil and big agriculture, there is far less nutrition in our food than there was 50 or 100 years ago. And that's assuming that people are eating fresh food—and not processed and fast food with empty calories. And even if you could get all of your nutrition from food, the fact is, some people need far higher levels of certain nutrients to be healthy, particularly those who are not well.

Vitamins and minerals are important catalysts for crucial bio-chemical reactions in our bodies, including in the muscles. When levels are too low, your metabolism is adversely affected. This can lead to fatigue, depression, and disease. In therapeutic doses, specific herbs, as well as vitamins and minerals, are helpful for musculoskeletal issues, like tightness, spasm, and inflammation, as well as for overall calm.

SUPPLEMENTS FOR MUSCLE TIGHTNESS AND SPASMS

- *Valeriana* (valerian), 200 to 300 milligrams every 4 hours as needed

- *Passiflora* (passion flower), 100 to 200 milligrams every 4 hours as needed

- Magnesium, 500 milligrams three times per day (magnesium glycinate or bisglycinate preferred)

- Calcium, 250 milligrams three times per day (calcium malate, glycinate, or citrate preferred)

- Proteolytic enzymes (trypsin, chymotrypsin, bromelain) 3 or 4 tablets four times per day between meals (*Do not take if you have an ulcer!*)

- Bioflavonoids (quercetin, hesperidin, rutin), 200 milligrams mixed bioflavonoids every 2 hours during acute phase

- Turmeric (*Curcuma longa*), 300 milligrams every 2 hours while swollen (standardized to 95 percent curcuminoids)

- Ginger, 200 milligrams every 2 hours while swollen (standardized to 5 percent gingerols)

- Boswellia, 400 milligrams every 2 hours while swollen (standardized to 70 percent boswellic acids)

- EPA-DHA combination (fish oil), 1,000 milligrams three times per day

SUPPLEMENTS FOR OVERALL CALM

- *Valeriana* (valerian), 200 to 400 milligrams once or twice per day as needed

- *Passiflora* (passion flower), 200 to 400 milligrams once or twice per day as needed

- Chamomile, 200 to 400 milligrams once or twice per day as needed

- *Melissa* (lemon balm), 200 to 400 milligrams once or twice per day as needed

Teas made from the calming herbs listed above can be a helpful addition. They can be used several times per day and prior to bedtime.

To conveniently order supplements for these purposes, check out the Fibro-Fix Structural packets and the products Myo-Fix, Inflamma-Fix, and Neuro-Fix at FibroFix.com or DrDavidBrady.com.

Stress Reduction Techniques

Please refer back to the Fibro-Fix Foundational Plan in Chapter 2 to revisit the whys and hows of using the gentle approaches below to reduce your stress and send your body and mind new signals of calm and comfort. If you have not yet found the time to take advantage of these approaches, I recommend that you do so now. They are an excellent complement to the more active forms of movement recommended in Chapter 2 and in this chapter.

- Guided imagery

- Meditation

- Yoga

- Reduction of social and occupational stressors

- Progressive muscle relaxation

- Moderate exercise (but do not overexercise)

Professional Support

I often refer patients who need additional help with musculoskeletal issues to physical therapists, chiropractors, massage therapists, practitioners of traditional Chinese medicine, acupuncturists, and herbalists. In this section, I'll go over what each of these practitioners does and how they can help you with your pain.

PHYSICAL THERAPY

Physical therapy, or physiotherapy (PT), supports the healing of injuries and physical impairments. PT also promotes mobility, function, and quality of life through examination, diagnosis, and intervention using a variety of strategies and techniques, including specific exercises; manual therapy and mobilization; mechanical devices such as traction; and physical agents like heat, cold, electricity, sound waves, radiation, prostheses, orthotics, and other interventions.

If you think back to Leon's story, these are the modalities that he needed to heal from his various injuries, not a hastily prescribed antidepressant.

Physical therapists use your history and a physical exam to arrive at a diagnosis and establish a plan for recovery. This might include treatment where movement and function are threatened by aging, injury, or disease. Movement is essential to maintaining health. A physical therapist can work with you to prevent the loss of mobility before it occurs. A physical therapist may also use lab tests, x-rays, CT scans, or MRIs.

Physical therapists practice in many settings, including privately owned therapy clinics; outpatient and health and wellness clinics; rehabilitation, skilled nursing, and extended-care facilities; private homes; schools; hospices; work environments; and fitness centers and sports-training facilities. They are licensed in all 50 states, and training is rigorous and consistent throughout the country. While physical therapists were trained at the bachelor's level only a decade or so ago, the degree level rose first to the master's and now to the doctoral level. While not all practicing therapists have doctoral degrees, as they may have completed their training before the degree level was raised, many have returned to complete their training as a doctor of physical therapy (DPT). Regardless, the training of a licensed physical therapist is something that generally can be relied upon with confidence.

However, while I greatly appreciate the work that many physical therapists do, they rely predominantly on rehabilitation exercises for strengthening and mobility. This can certainly be beneficial to people with musculoskeletal problems, especially those with orthopedic issues and those who are receiving poststroke therapy. But those with classic FM often cannot tolerate the level of exercise PT requires. And physical therapists are generally not trained to fully understand the issues at play in centrally mediated pain disorders, such as classic FM. (And they are certainly not alone in this fact.) Physical therapists also rely a great deal on passive modalities, including ultrasound and electrical muscle stimulation. And these modalities are generally not effective for those with classic FM, either, since the problem is not in the muscles, as you are now more than aware. These may help somewhat in the treatment of true musculoskeletal conditions but usually in a limited way.

What people with myofascial pain syndrome and trigger points really need is skilled, hands-on myofascial therapy. I find that physical therapists are generally not trained in this advanced hands-on technique, although some go on to do postgraduate seminars and workshops in myofascial therapy and become very proficient at it. This is the kind of physical therapist you need to find if you think you have a musculoskeletal issue and want to try PT.

There may be no health-care provider whose function is harder to summarize than a chiropractor. My own initial clinical training as a doctor of chiropractic (DC) has enabled me to see the many sides of this valuable, but oftentimes confusing, profession. Today's chiropractic physicians cover a broad range of treatment philosophies and practices. On one end of the spectrum are those who still cling to the original philosophies, and some may say dogma, of the profession—which suggests that the root of all disease and disharmony in the body stems from an improperly functioning nervous system that is receiving interference by small misalignments along the spine, called subluxations.

On the other side of the spectrum are chiropractors who act as "wide-scope natural" physicians, performing extensive diagnostic examinations and laboratory testing and prescribing elaborate therapeutic interventions that include the targeted use of vitamins, minerals, herbs, and lifestyle modifications, in addition to manual therapy. In fact, these types of chiropractors have paved the road in many ways for progressive holistic and integrative physicians of all types practicing today.

In practice, most chiropractors fall somewhere between the two extremes. But while the average chiropractor is likely to suggest a few vitamins and minerals, advocate dietary changes, and even the use of some herbs, most are focused mainly on musculoskeletal disorders, such as low-back pain, neck pain, and headache.

Adjustment, or spinal manipulation, remains the mainstay of chiropractic treatment. And there is no doubt that this is a powerful therapy in its own right. While it certainly can relieve many cases of back pain, neck pain, and headache, it may be doing more than that by removing the irritation of the sensitive nerves leaving the spinal column, which control critical functions all over the body. While there are numerous quality scientific studies that prove the efficacy, and even superiority, of chiropractic manipulation in treating many conditions, including low-back pain, reports of manipulation having positive effects on internal disorders (ranging from high blood pressure to colic) have historically remained mostly anecdotal in nature. Chiropractic adjustment can certainly help restore mobility and help those with various musculoskeletal conditions, but it has not proven to be an effective therapy for true centrally mediated pain disorders, like classic FM.

THE STORY OF CHIROPRACTIC

Founded in the late 19th century by Daniel David Palmer, of Davenport, Iowa, the chiropractic profession grew into a very popular organized health discipline that was becoming a threat to standard allopathic medicine. Colleges formed throughout the country, and many states licensed the profession due to pressure from those who had success with chiropractic treatment. However, a lot of early chiropractors were actually jailed for practicing medicine without a license before their states passed licensing laws. Unfortunately, the chiropractic profession became the victim of a decades-old slander and propaganda campaign by organized, political, allopathic (orthodox) medicine.

If you think this is a paranoid conspiracy tale, think again! In 1987 a federal court found the American Medical Association (AMA) guilty of conspiracy against the chiropractic profession, of racketeering, and of violating the federal RICO (Racketeer Influenced and Corrupt Organizations Act) and antitrust statutes (Wilk vs. AMA).[3] These laws were originally designed to prosecute organized crime! And while the chiropractic profession eventually won in the courtroom, the years of misinformation and outright slander took their toll, resulting in a lack of appreciation by the general public, as well as the medical community, for how extensively doctors of chiropractic are trained and how helpful they can be, especially with musculo-skeletal problems.

Nonetheless, alternative, complementary, holistic, and integrative medicine clinicians today owe a debt to the chiropractic profession. In many ways, it allowed the whole concept of an alternative to orthodox medicine to remain viable and in the public consciousness throughout the 1950s, 60s, 70s, and 80s, until the emergence of the modern natural and integrative medicine revolution. Several chiropractic colleges actually housed the only remaining programs in naturopathic medicine in the country throughout the first half of the 20th century, until enough interest was rekindled in natural medicine for independent accredited naturopathic medical colleges to emerge again in the 1970s and 80s.

I would recommend a chiropractor as an excellent choice when experiencing chronic musculoskeletal pain. I particularly recommend chiropractors who do not limit their practice only to adjustments or passive PT modalities but are also formally trained in and regularly use advanced soft-tissue methods—such as Active Release Technique (ART), Graston technique, Receptor-Tonus (Nimmo) technique, and/or myofascial release—in the treatment of myofascial pain syndrome and trigger points. If you are using, or considering using, a doctor of chiropractic to help you manage your problem with nutritional and herbal therapies, I suggest finding one with extensive postgraduate training in these areas. While the average chiropractic curriculum has substantially more in it about these therapies than the average conventional medical school program, it is still not enough to make one an expert. Ideally, you may want to look for a chiropractor who also has a board certification or master's degree in nutrition. Some letters you may see after a doctor's name who has advanced nutritional training include DACBN (diplomate of the American Clinical Board of Nutrition), DCBCN (diplomate of the Chiropractic Board of Clinical Nutrition), CNS (certified nutrition specialist), CCN (certified clinical nutritionist), and, optimally, an MS (master of science) in nutrition.

MASSAGE THERAPY

Who doesn't like a good massage? I think most people who have had a professional massage by a registered or licensed massage therapist (RMT, LMT) would agree it can be a very relaxing and often therapeutic experience. Massage has many benefits, ranging from actual reduction in muscle tightness to just plain old feeling better from pampering yourself. The benefits of actually dedicating for yourself a 30-, 60-, or even 90-minute block of time, combined with the action of having someone actually lay hands on you in a caring way, cannot be overstated.

Massage comes in various styles, ranging from Swedish massage, which is "light" and relaxing, to shiatsu and other deep forms of massage or pressure application meant to more aggressively treat particular muscular problem areas. Some therapists also train in advanced therapeutic techniques—such as myofascial release, St. John's technique, and others—to treat myofascial pain syndrome and trigger points. Some even train in a very aggressive treatment directed at the fascia called Rolfing, which may be perfect for some people with adhesions and musculoskeletal problems but is generally far too aggressive for anyone with classic FM.

If you're looking for a relaxing massage, these deeper methods may not be for you. However, if you have specific muscular problems, one of them may just fit the bill. It is up to you to clearly convey what your exact goals are for your massage to your massage therapist. If your muscular or joint problem seems severe, or if it is not steadily improving over time, I suggest a consultation with a licensed medical, naturopathic, or chiropractic doctor, or a physical therapist, for a more thorough evaluation.

The training requirements and laws governing licensure for massage therapists vary widely from state to state. Some states require comprehensive training and examination, while others don't require any. Always ask to see a therapist's license or registration to practice. Also consider using a therapist based on a personal referral.

One final point regarding massage therapists: Their training, along with the legal scope of their practice, is limited to massage. They do not have extensive training in the medical sciences, nor do they have the legal authority to diagnose disease. Unfortunately, I have had patients who were told by massage therapists that they had all sorts of problems, ranging from systemic yeast infections to calcium deficiencies to liver problems, all without the benefit of any form of objective diagnosis or laboratory testing. Numerous colleagues have reported similar experiences. Massage therapists are not qualified to diagnose whether or not you have FM.

Some massage therapists dole out advice on vitamins and herbal supplements, as well. I am not referring to giving basic recommendations, such as taking a multivitamin. I am talking about suggesting specific supplements or herbs for particular health problems. Unless the massage therapist has additional legitimate training and credentials in clinical nutrition, meaning an accredited academic degree, I would suggest seeing a qualified practitioner for nutritional or herbal guidance.

Unfortunately, the latest trend for some massage therapists is to emerge from a weekend seminar or two as "healers." Many study somewhat esoteric forms of hands-off energy therapy, including Reiki. While I do believe there are potential real benefits from various forms of energy-based therapies, this trend troubles me. In my opinion, those who are in this subset of massage therapists are over-stepping their bounds in regard to their training and legal authority in attempting to diagnose and treat patients for a whole host of real or fictional health conditions, basing their evaluations and advice on these diagnostic and treatment techniques with little to no evidence to support them.

I advise you find a well-trained massage therapist who just practices massage and who you have a good rapport with.

TRADITIONAL CHINESE MEDICINE

Any discussion of traditional Chinese medicine (TCM) is a difficult task in Western countries. These ancient modes of health care are based on entirely different cultural beliefs than those in the West. Westerners are schooled and raised in a society that accepts only the reductionist scientific biochemical model, while TCM is based on the accumulated empirical observation of patients over thousands of years.

Foundational to TCM are theories on the flow of life force and energy, or *chi*, within the body, including a balancing of the competitive energy forces of y*in* and y*ang*. The whole subject of proper energy flow, and its health ramifications within the body, has always been a difficult subject for Western medical scientists to comprehend. Since these theories and principles are very hard to quantify objectively in a laboratory, they have traditionally been rejected as hogwash (not a technical term!) by Western medicine. This, however, is changing rapidly, and bioenergetic medicine is now a hot new area in medical research. Many Western scientists are predicting that how energy is created, resonates, and flows within individual cells and throughout the body will represent the next great frontier in medicine. Only time will tell.

Traditional Chinese medicine has been practiced for over 5,000 years and was originally rooted in numerology and astrology. It predates Buddhism and Taoism, although some of the concepts of those spiritual paths have been interwoven with TCM. One Taoist concept that influences the practice of Chinese medicine is that there are no real causes or effects. According to Taoist thinking, things *just are,* with all things being predetermined and intertwined.

In Chinese medicine, treating a disease, as we do in Western medicine, occurs too late. Chinese medicine practitioners compare it to waiting until you are thirsty to start digging a well. The goal in Chinese medicine is to keep the patient balanced and healthy so disease does not ensue. Traditionally, Chinese physicians are paid only if a patient in their care *doesn't* get sick. A regular fee is paid to the physician as long as everyone in a family stays healthy. Think of this as the first true insurance policy ever written.

In the West, it is exactly the reverse. We are not excused from paying doctors or insurance premiums once we are sick and receiving medical care. In order to be cured, we pay *more* once we become sick. The sicker we become, the more we pay, and the more money is generated within the medical system. Where is the incentive to keep people well, and when they are ill, to get them better as quickly and completely as possible?

ACUPUNCTURE

While acupuncture was the first modality of Chinese medicine to gain Western attention, it is just one of the vast array of therapies within Asian medicine. Acupuncture involves the insertion of very thin needles into very specific spots on the body in an attempt to balance the flow of energy, or *chi,* as the Chinese refer to it. The needle stimulation either promotes energy flow that is blocked or reduces excess energy flowing in a specific area of the body. Using acupuncture on specific trigger points has also shown promise. Many people have found significant relief from this therapy.

Recently, rather than using needles, practitioners have begun to use fine streams of electrical current (electroacupuncture) or laser light to stimulate and move the energy and to treat trigger points. Although one who is well-trained can perform needle acupuncture with little or no pain, these new techniques make acupuncture more attractive to those with an aversion to needles.

For thousands of years, master practitioners of TCM have also used acupuncture to treat internal disorders of all types. In the West, its use is generally limited to reducing pain, particularly the pain associated with musculoskeletal problems, as well as to treating addictions, such as smoking and overeating.

In the East, TCM involves a long training usually done under the apprenticeship of a master practitioner. The treatment of internal or organ disorders is usually taught by the mentor only after the less-complicated pain-blocking and musculoskeletal techniques have been completely mastered by the student. Most Western-trained acupuncturists have not attained this level of expertise or received the comprehensive training needed to treat the more complicated internal-based disorders. However, this is changing with master's- and now doctoral-level training in acupuncture and TCM at accredited institutions in Western countries, including at my institution, the University of Bridgeport, through its Acupuncture Institute.

In the United States, acupuncture is regulated differently from state to state, with some states requiring higher levels of education than others. Commonly, it is practiced by licensed acupuncturists (LAc). Postgraduate acupuncture training is also available for medical, chiropractic, and naturopathic doctors. If you decide to try acupuncture, make sure you find a practitioner who has been properly trained. Physician basic training courses should be a minimum of 100 to 300 hours, while typical licensed acupuncturists have substantially more training than this and generally have a master's or now even a doctorate in TCM. If you decide to try acupuncture, make sure that, in addition to the practitioner being adequately trained, the facility is very clean and a brand-new, wrapped sterile needle is used for each insertion.

CHINESE HERBS

Many acupuncturists, and virtually all TCM doctors, use Chinese herbs to correct energy flow and provide balance within the systems of the body. The West began using Chinese medical herbs over 1,000 years ago. As the spice trade developed between the West and China, traders sought herbs to cure the great plagues of Europe. However, Chinese herbalism differs substantially from Western herbalism in that it uses a larger variety of herbs. Whole herbs that are not standardized to the level of any one particular active ingredient, as is the trend in Western herbalism, are generally used. And Chinese herbalists rarely use just one or two herbs. Typical Chinese herbal medicines contain a master, or "emperor," herb and many other helper, or "slave," herbs used in combination.

While Chinese medicine takes an entirely different approach to diagnosis and treatment than Western medicine, practitioners of TCM very often arrive at the same diagnosis as one another for a given complaint. This gives the TCM approach a high degree of what is known as interexaminer reliability. This essentially means the practitioners' diagnoses are consistent with one another. TCM diagnoses also tend to consistently correlate with Western medical diagnoses, even though the concept and names for the disorders may not be the same. This is very important, since both approaches are validated, even though they are entirely different from one another. In other words, there is more than one way to get there when it comes to diagnosis and treatment of human ailments. Remember, while we in the West tend to look at our high-tech, scientific-based medicine as the most valid and sophisticated medicine system, our system has been in existence for only a little more than 200 years. The Chinese system of medicine has been used, refined, and perfected for thousands of years. Things without value or validity do not tend to stick around and flourish for millennia!

Conclusion

A large array of tools can help with musculoskeletal issues, from stretches, massage, and physical therapy to chiropractic and acupuncture and Chinese medicine. Supplements and herbs can also help the musculoskeletal system to heal, reducing and even possibly eliminating symptoms.

The next chapter looks at how to begin the process of healing from functional disorders that are frequently misdiagnosed as fibromyalgia.

CHAPTER 6

THE FUNCTIONAL FIX

In the last chapter, you saw that the aches and pains of musculoskeletal issues can initially resemble the aches and pains of fibromyalgia. This chapter looks at how a variety of functional disorders can also masquerade as FM. A functional disorder is one that may not be severe enough to be recognized as a classically identified disease but represents a state of lower-level or suboptimal "function" in a metabolic process, organ, or system of the body. These functional disorders can result in a person feeling pain, fatigue, generalized intestinal distress, mild to moderate depression and anxiety, cognitive dysfunction, and other vague persistent symptoms. These kinds of functional issues often go undetected by physicians who have not been trained to look for them. This is the reason for the term *functional medicine*, which was discussed previously, and practitioners who have been trained in this model are versed in finding and resolving these kinds of issues. Left unaddressed, a functional issue can evolve into a clinical one—in other words, into a disease that conventional medicine attempts to address. Functional medicine, however, seeks to address subclinical problems way before a disease manifests.

I will show you how to find out if your chronic pain and fatigue are functional in nature. I will recommend tests that I use in my practice to identify these kinds of disorders. And I will describe what to do to lessen or eliminate functional pain and recapture your energy and vitality. If the results of the test you took in Chapter 3 indicated that you are not suffering from classic fibromyalgia, and if you suspect your issues are functional, pay close attention to the recommendations here.

Some common symptoms of functional issues include:

- Chronic airborne allergy
- Chronic infection
- Constipation
- Difficulty concentrating
- Extreme or persistent fatigue and low energy
- Facial puffiness
- Feeling cold all the time
- Food intolerance or sensitivity
- Frequent postnasal drip
- Hard time remembering things
- Inability to tolerate exercise
- Intestinal distress
- Joint pain
- Muscle cramps or aches
- Numbness or tingling
- Poor blood sugar control
- Weakness
- Unexplained weight gain

As you can see, this is a wide range of symptoms, and this represents only a partial list. Doctors often overlook common health signs like these because conventional medical training does not focus on ways to address the subtle dysfunctions that signify functional disorders. They don't show up on the traditionally trained clinician's radar.

Fortunately, this is the strength of functional medicine. I have years of training and experience that help me zero in on low-grade disorders that most commonly present as functional pain or fatigue. I frequently find functional disorders that other conventionally trained doctors have missed.

Functional Issues That Look Like FM

The functional problems most likely to cause widespread pain and fatigue include:

- Subtle functional hypothyroidism
- Effects of stress on the adrenal glands
- Gastrointestinal problems
- Mitochondrial dysfunction
- Nutritional deficiencies

- Chemical and food sensitivities
- Reactions to medication

Let's look at these one by one in more detail.

Subtle Functional Hypothyroidism

The thyroid gland consists of two lobes, one on either side of the trachea (windpipe) in the lower neck. A portion connecting the two lobes, called the isthmus, gives the entire gland an H-shaped appearance. The thyroid gland is responsible for synthesizing several hormones that have vast effects on overall body metabolism. The thyroid is unique among the endocrine glands in that large amounts of hormone are created and stored in the thyroid itself and then released very slowly. Iodine ingested from food and water is concentrated in the thyroid gland, where it combines with the amino acid tyrosine to create the thyroid hormones triiodothyronine (T3) and thyroxine (T4). The numbers 3 and 4 identify the number of iodine units in the hormone's structure. Generally speaking, lower levels of thyroid hormone will *slow* overall metabolism and energy, while higher levels will *increase* overall metabolism and energy. Thyroid-stimulating hormone (TSH), produced in the pituitary gland in the brain, influences all reactions controlling the formation of T3 and T4 (see Figure 6.1).

FIGURE 6.1 THYROID HORMONE CASCADE

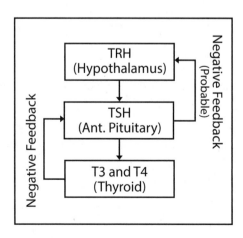

Having low thyroid function without actually having thyroid disease is very common, especially as we get older. Diminished thyroid function after age 40 occurs in about a quarter of the population. Because it's not an overt illness, it is sometimes called subtle or subclinical hypothyroidism. The symptoms are too minor to be declared an illness or disease according to standard medical measures. Yet, at the same time, they are too troublesome to allow you to feel really good. Symptoms of subtle functional hypothyroidism include:

- Cold hands and feet or a general feeling of being cold
- Constipation
- Dry, thinning hair
- Dry skin
- Facial puffiness
- Fatigue
- Gradual weight gain
- Mental sluggishness
- Muscle and joint achiness
- Thinning of the outer third of the eyebrows

You can see why many with suboptimal thyroid function can be easily misdiagnosed as having fibromyalgia.

In addition to these symptoms, people with a functional hypothyroid condition may experience:

- Carpal tunnel syndrome
- Chronic infections
- Frequent postnasal drip
- High blood sugar
- High cholesterol
- Inability to tolerate exercise
- Numbness/tingling
- Weakness

Thyroid function laboratory tests should be routinely performed in patients who present with complaints of widespread pain and fatigue in order to rule out significant or obvious hypothyroidism as the cause of these symptoms. These tests should include thyroperoxidase antibodies and thyroglobulin antibodies tests to screen for cases of autoimmune thyroid conditions, such as Graves' disease and Hashimoto's thyroiditis. Even when standard lab values are within the normal ranges, subtle variations of thyroid dysfunction should be considered.

Many cases of hypothyroidism will respond well to the use of common hormone replacement medications, such as Synthroid, Levothroid, or Levoxyl. However, these medications contain only a synthetic version of the hormone thyroxine (T4). The problem here is that to be useful, T4 (the comparatively inactive "storage" hormone) must be converted to T3, and some people are unable to do this very well. Instead, they produce too little of the active T3 and too much of the mainly inactive form of the T3 hormone, known as reverse T3, or rT3. (See Figure 6.2.) This condition is sometimes referred to as euthyroid sick syndrome, low T3 syndrome, or thyroid hormone peripheral conversion disorder. In these situations, people often do not feel relief of their symptoms when placed on synthetic T4 alone.

FIGURE 6.2 THYROID HORMONE CONVERSION

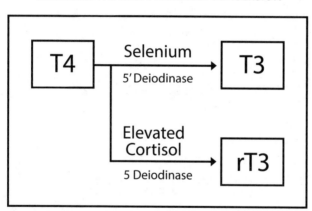

These types of thyroid dysfunction are subtler than the kinds of problems conventional family doctors, and even most endocrinologists, screen for. One possible reason for these conversion problems may be elevated cortisol levels due to acute or long-term stress. Cortisol, an adrenal hormone, is known to negatively affect the enzyme that converts T4 to active T3, called 5'-deiodinase. The use of combinations of T4 and T3 (for example, the natural, porcine-derived Armour Thyroid and Nature-Throid, or the combination of the synthetic medications Synthroid and Cytomel) are gaining popularity with many physicians attempting to help people with this issue. However, too often, conventional doctors will tell people that their thyroid function is just fine. Often that is just not so.

In my view, doctors should pay close attention to *all* clinical symptoms, measure core temperature, and use comprehensive thyroid laboratory testing to gain a complete and accurate picture of thyroid function. If laboratory tests show that you are in the lower part of the normal range for both the total and free forms of the T3 and T4 hormones—or if your TSH results are in the upper part of the normal range—and if you also have many clinical symptoms of low thyroid function, a functional-medicine physician will typically consider a trial of comprehensive thyroid hormone treatment.

As I mentioned earlier, functional hypothyroidism can also be due to an autoimmune disorder known as Hashimoto's disease, in which the immune system attacks the thyroid gland. Hashimoto's can initially cause hyperthyroidism, but will eventually result in exhaustion of the thyroid due to tissue damage to the gland and an inability to produce an

THYROID HORMONE MARKERS

Here's what you'll learn from a thyroid panel. High levels of thyroid-stimulating hormone (TSH) indicate an underactive thyroid. In addition, the panel also separately tests triiodothyronine (T3) and thyroxine (T4) levels. T4 and T3 each exist in two forms: either bound to proteins in the blood, where they are kept in reserve for later use, or "free" (known as FT3 and FT4) and immediately available to enter body tissues wherever needed to upregulate metabolism. High levels of T4 and/or T3 suggest hyperthyroidism, while low levels of either T4 and/or T3 suggest hypothyroidism. In some cases of hyperthyroidism, FT4 is normal yet FT3 is elevated. Attention must be paid to the level of the free hormones, particularly free T3, for an accurate picture of what is happening metabolically. Even a free T3 in the lower level of the "normal" range can indicate suboptimal thyroid function if clinical symptoms and complaints typical of hypothyroidism are also present. However, if your doctor does not test this, you will simply never know.

adequate amount of thyroid hormone. Functional hypothyroidism may also occur when, over a long period of time, the body has sent out too many false alarms to initiate the fight-or-flight response due to stress. These false alarms arouse the adrenals and thyroid to action. This is why it's important to evaluate the status and functioning of the adrenal glands along with the thyroid.

In my experience, undiagnosed thyroid issues are one of the prime reasons for complaints of fatigue, achiness, and cognitive dysfunction—and the eventual misdiagnosis of FM—particularly in women.

Donna's Story

After complaints of general pain and achiness, fatigue, insomnia, unrefreshing sleep, and mild depression, Donna was diagnosed with FM by her family doctor. He put her on an SNRI antidepressant called venlafaxine (Effexor) and zolpidem tartrate (Ambien), a gamma-aminobutyric acid (GABA) receptor agonist, to help her sleep. For people with classic FM, these medications can be helpful, but all they seemed to do for Donna was to make her feel more groggy and spacey, without any real improvement in her symptoms. Although she didn't realize it at the time, this was one important clue that Donna did *not* have classic FM. Hoping that there might be another road to recovery, Donna attended a teleseminar I presented. She decided to make an appointment and came to my office seeking alternative approaches.

I began by ordering a number of tests that would show how well various bodily functions were working. These included:

☐ **Blood chemistry:** This test is used to assess overall function of the major organs and systems of the body, but it is designed to find overt disease not optimal "function."

☐ **Complete blood count (CBC):** The CBC is used to determine an individual's general health by detecting the presence of anemia, infection, inflammation, bleeding disorders, and many other conditions (such as blood-based cancers, like leukemia and lymphomas).

☐ **Iron studies:** This involves running three different tests (serum iron, serum ferritin, and percent iron saturation) that together evaluate the levels of iron in the bloodstream and various tissues. Low levels of iron are associated with a specific form of anemia known as microcytic anemia, which can result in the red blood cells being unable to efficiently carry oxygen. And this can cause metabolic dysfunctions, especially in the production of energy, making you fatigued and leaving you with achy muscles.

- **Erythrocyte sedimentation rate (ESR):** This is a simple, inexpensive test that is used to detect systemic, or body-wide, inflammation. ESR is said to be "nonspecific" because, while an elevated result indicates inflammation, the test does not tell the practitioner where the inflammation is or what is causing it.

- **C-reactive protein (CRP):** Within a few hours of a tissue injury, infection, or other source of inflammation, the liver releases CRP into the blood. This test for CRP can be used together with symptoms and other tests to help determine if an acute or chronic inflammatory condition exists.

- **Thyroid panel:** The thyroid panel tests for TSH, various forms of the T4 and T3 hormones, and thyroid-related autoantibodies to screen for autoimmune diseases of the thyroid, like Hashimoto's and Graves' disease.

Donna's lab tests showed normal blood chemistry, CBC, and iron studies, and she was negative for certain key inflammatory markers (i.e., the ESR and CRP tests). Her thyroid panel was also technically normal, but on closer examination of the hormone levels, it became clear that there were certain imbalances, leading to suboptimal function.

Her total and free T3 levels were at the very bottom of the normal range, while her total and free T4 levels were also suboptimal, though better than the T3 levels. Her TSH was still in the normal range but in the very high part of the range. In sum, the amount of active thyroid hormone she was getting was low, and her body was asking for more.

Another test that I frequently order for my patients is the simple and affordable organic acids test (OAT). This can often reveal issues in the biochemistry of energy production, which accompany low or suboptimal thyroid drive. When Donna's test results came in, they revealed some inefficiencies in energy production. They also showed that Donna was not effectively detoxifying chemicals and hormones that needed to be cleared from her body. Her serotonin metabolite (5-HIAA) was also low, but her stress hormone (catecholamine) metabolites were normal, which indicated a possible deficiency in her ability to manufacture an optimal amount of the important neurotransmitter hormone serotonin. However, she did not have the anxiety and insomnia typically seen in classic FM patients.

Taken all together, these tests revealed to me that Donna mainly had subtle functional hypothyroidism due to suboptimal thyroid hormone production as well as poor thyroid hormone conversion of T4 to T3. Her unique biochemistry and metabolism also needed some tweaking, including increasing her ability to generate energy in the cells, to detoxify waste products, and to produce serotonin.

Donna's Treatment Plan

At my urging, Donna went on the 21-day Fibro-Fix Foundational Plan. She began taking CoQ10, L-carnitine, D-ribose, and B-complex vitamins (for energy and mitochondrial metabolism support). For thyroid support, she began taking Nature-Throid, which supplies both the T3 and T4 hormones; a supplement containing selenium, N-acetyl tyrosine, and iodine to support thyroid hormone production and conversion; and a bit of 5-HTP for better serotonin production.

Follow-up thyroid lab tests performed 4 weeks later guided me in adjusting the dosage to keep Donna in the upper 50 percent of all thyroid hormone ranges, but never above the normal range. For her occasional sleep issues, she began taking 3 milligrams of sustained-release melatonin just prior to bedtime.

After 30 days, Donna showed a 75 percent improvement in all symptoms (fatigue, achiness, insomnia, and unrefreshing sleep). After 60 days, her symptoms disappeared. And a 6-month follow-up showed that her condition had not returned.

Getting the thyroid working optimally is essential. If it's not working well, almost nothing else will. It's something I pay as much attention to in my practice as anything else with chronically ill patients. Therefore, if you are not currently working with a doctor who is trained in integrative medicine, and even more specifically in functional medicine, and you think you may have an issue with your thyroid, please find a physician who will give you a comprehensive thyroid function evaluation. If you can't come to my practice in Connecticut, you may want to consult the Additional Resources section of this book (page 259) for some options on how to find a provider trained in the functional-medicine approach.

To learn more about functional hypothyroid disorders, please visit DrDavidBrady.com. To conveniently order supplements for this purpose, including Thyro-Fix, visit FibroFix.com.

Effects of Stress on the Adrenal Glands

In all people complaining of fatigue, doctors should evaluate adrenal gland function. Increases in the levels of catecholamines, the fight-or-flight stress hormones (often called adrenaline) produced by the adrenal glands, cause increases in sympathetic nervous system activity. As you may remember, overactivation of the sympathetic nervous system has been associated with classic FM (see page 77), along with other problems misdiagnosed as FM. Levels of cortisol, another stress hormone produced by the adrenal glands, should also be assessed when screening for adrenal dysfunction. The pattern of low cortisol and elevated catecholamines is common in FM and has also been associated with post-traumatic stress disorder. This may explain the emergence of FM in people who have undergone significant stress, life-altering events, abuse, or trauma.

The pattern of these hormones in an individual can be assessed using the organic acids test for the catecholamines and the adrenal stress profile/index salivary tests for cortisol. Both tests are discussed in detail later in the chapter. For people with this classic pattern of low cortisol and elevated catecholamines, psychological counseling and stress-reducing lifestyle modifications are extremely important.

For supplements for balancing adrenal function, see Chapter 4, page 104.

Gastrointestinal Problems

The gastrointestinal problems that are commonly associated with FM are irritable bowel syndrome and small intestinal bacteria overgrowth (SIBO).

IRRITABLE BOWEL SYNDROME

The chronic functional bowel disorder known as irritable bowel syndrome (IBS) affects approximately 11 to 14 percent of the population. It's a condition with multiple causes and features, including:

- Abnormal brain-gut interaction

- Altered bowel microbial balance (dysbiosis)

- Altered motility (movement of food through the intestines)

- Gut immune hyperactivation

- Gut inflammation

- Intestinal hypersensitivity

IBS is characterized by an exaggerated perception of pain in the gut (hyperalgesia)—an effect similar to those seen in the muscles and soft tissues with the central hypersensitivity of classic fibromyalgia, which I've already discussed (see page 77). Gut hypersensitivity, measured by decreased tolerance for gut distension (stretching), is considered a biological marker of IBS.

Many research studies have demonstrated a common association (or comorbidity)—ranging from 30 to over 80 percent—between IBS and classic FM. However, since the commonly used diagnostic criteria for FM *includes* IBS, the relationship between these syndromes is difficult to analyze fully and accurately. For example, the fact that both IBS and FM are much more common in women has led some researchers to suggest that IBS in women is due mainly to them having FM. However, while many women suffering from classic FM *do* have IBS, many women do not meet the criteria for classic FM but still have IBS. And this can contribute to the misdiagnosis of FM.

Besides gut complaints, people with IBS also have many other symptoms—like depression, anxiety, and insomnia—that are consistent with the central sensitization states seen in global pain disorders like classic FM. This suggests not only co-existence between IBS and FM in many people but also that they may be caused by some of the same mechanisms.

In summary, the dysfunctions in the central nervous system that are part of classic FM are virtually the same as the dysfunctions seen in the enteric nervous system (the nervous system of the intestines) in IBS. This includes the major role of the neurotransmitter serotonin in both disorders. In fact, several of the prescription medications that are used to treat IBS work by binding to and modulating the specific serotonin receptors located in the gut tissues.

Laboratory analysis useful in assessing the gastrointestinal environment and individual reactions to foods, which are key to the resolution of IBS symptoms, include stool analysis and food sensitivity testing.

Stool Analysis. I use the latest molecular-based technology, which looks for the DNA or genes of organisms—including bacteria, viruses, fungi, yeast, and parasites—present in the intestines. This test is called the GI-MAP, a fitting name, since this test essentially maps a person's individual gut environment to determine how many good (beneficial), bad (pathogenic), and opportunistic organisms are growing in the gut. This allows the treating doctor to support the intestinal environment by eradicating any bad organisms, fostering the growth of beneficial organisms, and rebalancing the environment for optimal GI function. For more information on the GI-MAP test, and to share it with your doctor or health-care provider, please visit DiagnosticSolutionsLab.com.

Food Sensitivity Testing. Several methods for testing food intolerance or food sensitivities are available. The method I have always found to be the most comprehensive is the ALCAT test (ALCAT.com). This test requires a blood sample. Rather than checking only for IgE and/or IgG antibodies formed in response to particular food proteins, as most food allergy and sensitivity tests do, the ALCAT test analyzes minute changes that occur to immune system cells called leukocytes (white blood cells), as well as platelets and plasma proteins, prior to and after the blood is exposed to specific food substances. (See Figure 6.3.)

However, the ALCAT test will not detect IgE reactions, which generally involve immediate, and potentially life-threatening, anaphylactic reactions to foods. But because these reactions are so immediate, lab testing is often not required. A person having such a reaction can easily tell what the offending food was. Of course, there do exist standard commercial lab tests to determine these kinds of reactions, and allergists routinely perform these if a food allergy of this type is suspected. Skin-prick testing with the offending food is also commonly performed and can detect these types of immediate reactions, but it can't find the delayed-sensitivity reactions, immune activation, and inflammation response to foods that the ALCAT test can find.

FIGURE 6.3 CHANGES TO THE IMMUNE SYSTEM
UPON EXPOSURE TO FOODS

Pre-antigen exposure

Post-antigen exposure

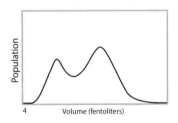

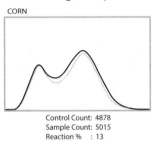

Source: Cell Science Systems/ALCAT, Deerfield Beach, FL. Used with permission.

Completing a food sensitivity test and using what you learn to eliminate those foods from your diet can greatly reduce the symptoms of IBS (as well as other symptoms common to people diagnosed either correctly or incorrectly with FM). Over time, as your digestive function and gastrointestinal health improve, you can gradually reintroduce many of the foods you eliminated.

SMALL INTESTINAL BACTERIAL OVERGROWTH

Patients with classic FM frequently have nonspecific gut complaints similar to those with a disorder known as small intestinal bacterial overgrowth (SIBO). SIBO is a condition in which many of the bacteria that normally grow in the intestines, mainly the colon (large intestine), overgrow further up in the small intestine. There is a growing body of medical evidence suggesting that SIBO may even play a significant role in a wide range of other gastrointestinal disorders, including inflammatory bowel diseases, such as Crohn's disease and colitis.

There is also emerging evidence in the medical research that suggests that there is micro-inflammation within the brain in those with classic FM. It is also theorized that this may be due, at least in part, to bacterial endotoxins (the chemicals excreted by the abnormal levels and sometimes unhealthy types of bacteria overgrowing in the intestines of people suffering from global pain and fatigue syndromes). These bacteria can produce an environment that fosters leaky gut syndrome and the activation of the immune system and inflammation-producing cytokines. These chemicals, including lipopolysaccharides produced by the bacteria, activate TLR4 (toll-like receptor-4) of the microglial cells of the brain, producing brain inflammation and alterations in neurochemistry and nerve transmission, which may lead to global pain and the central sensitivity syndrome symptoms associated with classic FM. Other toxins associated with these overgrowing bacteria can negatively affect the mitochondria within the cells responsible for producing energy, resulting in persistent fatigue.

Common symptoms of SIBO include gas, bloating, and distension of the abdomen, especially after eating high-starch or carbohydrate-rich foods, such as bread, potatoes, pasta, and rice. The most commonly used laboratory method to confirm SIBO is a lactulose hydrogen and methane breath test, which looks for evidence of the excessive gas generated by these overgrowing bacteria when they ferment sugars and starches in the diet.

Many people are able to eradicate SIBO with antibiotic therapy, improving both GI symptoms and the general symptoms of pain, fatigue, and sleeplessness. The antibiotic rifaximin (Xifaxan) acts locally in the intestines with negligible absorption into the body, minimal side effects, and a broad-spectrum of activity against the common bacteria responsible for most cases of SIBO, resulting in eradication in up to 70 percent of cases. Rifaximin also acts against *Clostridium difficile,* a bacteria commonly associated with causing diarrhea.

However, other options for treating SIBO are important to consider as rifaximin is very expensive, often not available, and frequently not covered by insurance. Other options include the antibiotics neomycin (a low-cost nonabsorbable antibiotic) and norfloxacin. Natural GI antimicrobials can also be very effective in treating SIBO, as well as other gastrointestinal infections. Studies by Gerard E. Mullin, MD, an integrative gastroenterologist and nutritionist at Johns Hopkins Hospital, and his colleagues have demonstrated that using natural botanical and volatile oils can be as effective, and sometimes more effective, than rifaximin

THE VALUE OF FUNCTIONAL EVALUATION METHODS

Recently, Cynthia, a friend of a friend, experienced a tremendous craving for salt. She reported that she added 6 teaspoons of table salt to her food over the course of the day. Her conventional doctors saw no problem with this highly unusual level of salt consumption because her blood pressure was normal. They took no steps to find out the reasons for this sudden craving, nor did they consider what the long-term effects of high salt consumption might be. From their perspectives, they would only raise a red flag *after* Cynthia had developed measurable high blood pressure.

This is an example of overreliance on one test (the blood pressure reading) due to lack of knowledge of other tests that reveal functional imbalances. Often, conventional doctors ignore major opportunities for timely health interventions because they don't know about (or choose to use) many of these helpful tests.

When your body is not functionally well or is producing a novel symptom (like Cynthia's salt craving), it's not always possible for either you or your doctor to accurately guess what precisely isn't working. In Cynthia's case, her work involved frequent and unexpected last-minute travel. The salt craving was the result of adrenal dysfunction and exhaustion due to stress, resulting in lower-than-normal aldosterone production. Aldosterone is a hormone produced by the adrenal glands that governs salt reuptake/retention by the kidneys.

Doctors use tests to look into key functional areas to figure out what is not working, and many such tests have been developed. Functional medicine doctors like me rely upon these assessments to see what is going on inside your body and to correct it both before (and even after) problems have developed.

Laboratory testing of metabolic function may include detecting:

- ☐ Excessive levels of body oxidative stress
- ☐ Inefficient cellular energy production
- ☐ Lowered detoxification ability
- ☐ Suboptimal levels of vitamins and minerals

and other prescription antibiotics, with fewer side effects.[1] These natural agents include substances such as:

- *Artemisia annua* (wormwood)
- Berberine-containing botanicals (such as barberry, officially known as *Berberis vulgaris*)
- Caprylic acid
- Grapefruit and other citrus seed extracts
- *Juglans nigra* (black walnut)
- Oil of oregano

For guidance on testing and the appropriate use of antibiotic, or natural antimicrobial, therapy for IBS or SIBO, please consult with a functional or integrative medicine provider familiar with these approaches.

Mitochondrial Dysfunction

Mitochondrial dysfunction is a disorder of the tiny energy producing "factories" that are present within every cell in your body, except for your red blood cells. These little power plants generate 95 percent of your body's energy by converting oxygen and food molecules into the body's fuel, adenosine triphosphate (or ATP), as shown in Figure 6.4. Your mitochondria also speed up wound healing and recovery.

In a number of ways, mitochondria behave like bacteria, from which they are probably derived. They are constantly dividing in two through a process called biogenesis, changing their shape, and fusing with each other. Using a muscle results in more mitochondria being created in that muscle. But if the mitochondria are dysfunctional, they can't keep up with your energy demand—like a busy restaurant that's running out of food with a room full of waiting customers. This is why your mitochondrial health is strongly tied to your fitness, and even your longevity.

Mitochondria are particularly susceptible to damage from oxidative stress. And mitochondrial dysfunction, with its associated ATP deficiency, is related to a host of diseases, including chronic fatigue syndrome, degenerative neurological disorders, cardiovascular disease, obesity, and even diabetes.

FIGURE 6.4 CELLULAR ENERGY PRODUCTION

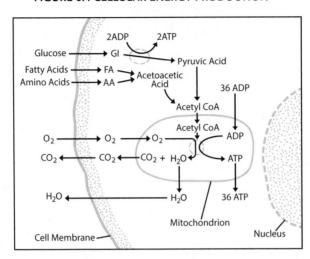

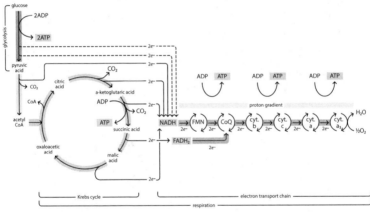

Mitochondrial dysfunction is connected to degenerative disorders, such as:

- Alzheimer's
- Amyotrophic lateral sclerosis
- Cardiovascular disease
- Diabetes
- Heart attack

- Multiple sclerosis
- Obesity
- Parkinson's
- Peripheral vascular disease
- Stroke

(continued on page 179)

A TESTING GUIDE FOR YOUR
HEALTH-CARE PROVIDER

Here is a guide that you can bring to your doctor on some of the most useful functional tests currently available.

Organic Acids Test

One of the most comprehensive methods is known as organic acids test (OAT).[2] Comprehensive urinary OAT panels are now available from several commercial laboratories. (At the end of this sidebar, I list the URLs of some labs that commonly provide these services to the integrative and functional-medicine community.) Elevated levels of specific organic acids may indicate a functional block or inhibition of specific metabolic pathways due to a person's unique inherited enzyme deficits, their production of structurally damaged or deranged enzymes, and/or their nutrient insufficiencies.

Results from the organic acids test that are pertinent to treating those misdiagnosed with FM—and often those diagnosed correctly with classic FM—include the following:

☐ Elevated urinary levels of malate, fumarate, succinate, alpha-ketoglutarate, hydroxymethylglutarate, and other Krebs cycle (the biochemical pathways responsible for the bulk of energy production in the body) intermediates may indicate CoQ10, B-vitamin, and/or magnesium deficiency or other issues related to mitochondrial function and energy production. Clinical correlations include fatigue and muscle ache, and interventions should include increased intake, through alteration of diet and/or supplementation, of CoQ10, B vitamins, magnesium, and other critical nutrient cofactors.

☐ Elevations in catecholamine metabolites, such as vanilmandelate and/or homovanillate, can be indicative of the typical sympathetic compensation pattern and hypervigilance observed in classic FM, irritable bowel syndrome, and post-traumatic stress disorder (see Figure 6.5). Clinical correlations include anxiety, panic attacks, insomnia, and overall signs of hypervigilance. Intervention may include cognitive behavioral therapy (for example, progressive muscle relaxation, meditation, prayer, yoga, tai chi, and qigong), other relaxation practices, and the use of adaptogenic botanicals/herbs and calming neurotransmitter precursors as outlined in Chapter 4.

FIGURE 6.5 CATECHOLAMINE PRODUCTION AND METABOLISM

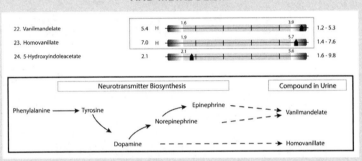

Source: J. A. Bralley and R. S. Lord, eds., Laboratory Evaluations for Integrative and Functional Medicine, 2nd ed., chapter 6, (Asheville, NC: Metametrix Institute-Genova Diagnostics, 2008). Used with permission.

☐ Deficiency of 5-hydroxyindoleacetate (5-HIAA) is indicative of reduction in total body serotonin (5-HT) production—which may correlate with increased pain perception, mild depression, irritable bowel syndrome (IBS), and insomnia—and serves as a possible indicator for the use of prescription or natural serotonin modulators as outlined in Chapter 4 (also see Figure 6.6). Abnormalities of the kynurenine-quinolinate pathway of tryptophan metabolism can be seen on the test, as well, which is important as this can lead to alterations in pain perception via NMDA (N-methyl-D-aspartate) receptor activation. Elevations in these markers may indicate the

(continued)

need for treatment of any underlying degenerative/inflammatory neurological conditions. Reduction of systemic inflammation with omega-3 fatty acid (EPA-DHA from fish oil) therapy is also potentially indicated.

FIGURE 6.6 SEROTONIN PRODUCTION AND METABOLISM

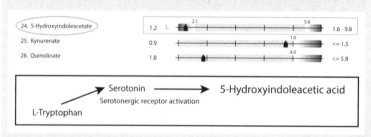

Source: J. A. Bralley and R. S. Lord, eds., Laboratory Evaluations for Integrative and Functional Medicine, 2nd ed., chapter 6, (Asheville, NC: Metametrix Institute-Genova Diagnostics, 2008). Used with permission.

☐ The status of B vitamins, carnitine, and other nutrients critical to energy production can also be evaluated through OAT. Clinical correlations include fatigue and muscle ache, and dietary changes and/or supplementation can be initiated as required.

☐ Increased recovery of methylmalonate and formiminoglutamate indicates an insufficiency of vitamin B_{12} and folate, respectively, potentially resulting in anemia and suboptimal methylation and genetic expression. In those with elevations in either of these markers, increased intake of methylated folate and/or B_{12} can be initiated through dietary changes and/or supplementation.

☐ Elevated levels of various metabolic by-products of opportunistic or pathogenic gastrointestinal organisms is indicative of a dysbiotic state and/or SIBO, with D-arabinitol specifically suggestive of Candida species yeast overgrowth. Clinical correlations include bloating, cramping, and excessive flatulence, especially after eating starches and carbohydrate-rich foods, and interventions may include prescription or natural antimicrobial therapy, as discussed previously in the section on SIBO.

Adrenal Stress Profile/Index

The adrenal stress profile/index (ASP/ASI), depending on the lab used, is a useful noninvasive (no blood test required) salivary hormone test that evaluates bioactive levels of the body's important stress hormones, cortisol and DHEA (dehydroepiandrosterone). This test is useful for uncovering biochemical imbalances underlying anxiety, depression, fibromyalgia, chronic fatigue syndrome, obesity, blood sugar abnormalities, and a host of other conditions.

These hormone tests generally examine four saliva samples collected over a 24-hour period for levels of cortisol and one test for DHEA. The human adrenal glands do not secrete cortisol at a constant level throughout the day. Cortisol is actually released in a cycle, with the highest value in the morning and the lowest value at night, when functioning properly. This 24-hour cycle is called the circadian rhythm. Aberrations in the levels of this hormone throughout the day can be indicative of prolonged stress and maladaptation of the adrenal glands in response to stressful situations and stimuli. As you can see from Figure 6.7—which contains actual lab results from one of my patients— the levels here are a bit too high in the morning and too low at night. This corresponds to the significant ongoing stress, and resulting exhaustion, this patient was actually experiencing, revealing again that what people experience can often be measured and tracked.

Based on your personal results, a knowledgeable health-care provider can determine what types of therapies may be useful to balance your stress response and return you to a more vibrant state of health. Many suggestions were made in the previous discussions on adrenal health, such as the use of adaptogenic botanicals/herbals and calming neurotransmitter precursors (discussed in Chapter 4). Proper and consistent sleep hygiene is also very important in establishing or

(continued)

FIGURE 6.7 ADRENAL STRESS INDEX/PROFILE SAMPLE TEST RESULT

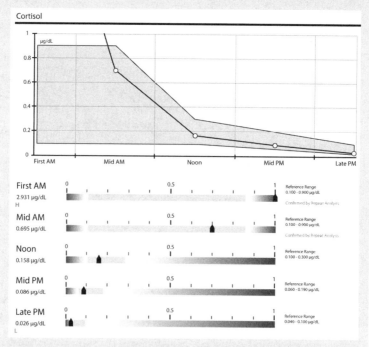

Source: Source: Cell Science Systems/ALCAT, Deerfield Beach, FL. Used with permission.

reinforcing a healthy 24-hour circadian rhythm. This includes consistently getting to bed early enough (generally not after 10 p.m. or 11 p.m.), waking at a typical time (generally between 7 a.m. and 8 a.m.), and maintaining a quality sleep environment (such as a dark and quiet room free of pets or small children).

The OAT and ASP/ASI are generally repeated after 2 to 4 months to assess improvement in metabolic and adrenal function in areas found to be suboptimal during initial testing and to help in altering and refining the treatment approach.

To learn more about the OAT test, visit GreatPlainsLaboratory.com or GDX.net, and to learn more about the ASP/ASI, please visit CellScienceSystems.com, DiagnosTechs.com, and GDX.net.

Some mitochondrial dysfunction—as much as 15 percent—is caused by mutations in cell DNA. Mitochondria also deteriorate with age. As they decline, the cells become damaged and starved for energy, causing them to function less efficiently. Many investigators suspect that the reason a calorie-restricted diet slows aging is that it lowers free radical production and therefore lessens damage to the mitochondria. So there are many benefits to increased mitochondrial biogenesis and increased ATP, including the lessening of age-related deterioration and an increase in energy levels, ability to exercise, cognitive function, and life span.

Christine's Story

Christine, 36 years old, was happily married to a supportive husband and had two children. Her own childhood, growing up in Taiwan, was loving and safe. There was no history of anxiety or depression. She suffered from generalized achiness, long-standing fatigue, and chronic constipation alternating with diarrhea but no intestinal cramping, distension, or bloating.

Christine reported that she had a hard time thinking clearly, remembering things, and staying on-task. She said she had been experiencing some body-wide muscle tenderness and pain. My exam of major muscle groups confirmed that there was muscle achiness and tenderness but no exaggerated pain responses to digital pressure. Her muscles generally lacked spasticity, and there were only a couple of myofascial trigger points noted in the upper shoulder/trap muscles, probably due to normal stress and postural distortions. Nor was there any joint swelling or pain. As you learned in the prior chapter, had these been present to a greater extent, they might have indicated a musculoskeletal problem. Since that was not the case with Christine, I continued to investigate.

Christine's vital signs, her heart, lung, and thyroid, were normal on examination. And an orthopedic and neurological exam failed to reveal any issues.

Christine's lab tests were normal for thyroid, iron, inflammation, and autoimmune markers. However, an organic acid test revealed significant problems with the biochemistry of energy production. There was clearly difficulty in aerobic metabolism (using oxygen in the mitochondria) and an overreliance on anaerobic metabolism (non-oxygen-dependent pathways outside of the mitochondria) to produce energy. This kind of metabolism results in far less energy output and the accumulation of acidic waste products, such as lactic acid. On an ongoing basis, this makes the muscles tender and sore, causes overall energy depletion and fatigue, and results in cognitive dysfunction (since the brain requires a great deal of energy).

Stool analysis using molecular DNA technology to map the GI microbial population showed no pathogenic or imbalanced flora. But Christine's levels of beneficial bacteria—the healthy gut microbes that promote good digestion and immunity—were suboptimal. Food sensitivity testing revealed multiple food sensitivities, including a sensitivity to whey and casein proteins in dairy.

Christine went on the 21-day Fibro-Fix Foundational Plan, which eliminates inflammatory, allergenic, and dairy-based foods. She began taking CoQ10, L-carnitine, D-ribose, and B-complex vitamins for energy and mitochondrial metabolism support, along with probiotics. For constipation, she began taking magnesium citrate and fiber powder in the morning.

After 30 days, she showed an improvement in all symptoms. After 60 days, there was an approximately 90 percent improvement in all symptoms. When I saw her for a 6-month follow-up, she had excellent energy and vitality, no muscle tenderness, and no constipation.

Nutritional Deficiencies

Several nutritional deficiencies are commonly observed in patients with ongoing fatigue and widespread tenderness, regardless of whether they have classic FM or there are other functional reasons for these symptoms.

COQ10 AND CARNITINE

Coenzyme Q10 (CoQ10) and carnitine are both absolutely critical for the production of energy in the cells, proper brain and muscle function, and an overall optimal metabolism.

CoQ10—an oil-soluble, vitamin-like substance—is one of the raw materials your mitochondria need to make ATP.[3] The organs of your body that require the most energy—your heart, liver, and kidneys—have the most CoQ10. Mutations in the genes required for the biosynthesis of CoQ10 can cause shortages or deficiencies. If your CoQ10 is low, it may be because your body is not making enough of it. Chronic illness may also affect CoQ10 levels.[4] One of the most prescribed classes of medications today, known as the statins, used to lower cholesterol levels, is notorious for also lowering the body's production of CoQ10.[5] This is particularly true when they are used at higher doses (for example, Lipitor at 40 milligrams per day) and a big reason why many people on these medications complain of fatigue and muscle achiness.

If you are experiencing fatigue and muscle achiness while taking statin medications, I strongly suggest you work with your prescribing doctor to safely lower the dose while you implement alternate methods to modify your cardiovascular risk and lower your LDL cholesterol. These strategies may include dietary changes (like going on a healthy diet of lean proteins and fresh vegetables, fruits, and fibers) and the use of natural agents known to favorably alter lipid profiles, such as niacin, red yeast rice, and bergamot (*Citrus bergamia risso*), an extract from a citrus plant that grows almost exclusively in the narrow coastal Calabria region in southern Italy.

Too little carnitine affects the availability of fatty acids in the mitochondria, which can cause them to produce too little ATP. Carnitine is necessary as a "shuttle" substance to carry fats into the mitochondria to burn as energy and produce ATP. While the body can produce carnitine from the amino acids lysine and methionine, derived from protein food sources, carnitine is also derived directly from animal protein. Since animals maintain carnitine in their muscle tissue, when that tissue is eaten as meat, the carnitine is acquired. This is why it's generally even more critical that vegetarians and vegans have their carnitine levels assessed when fatigue and muscle ache are experienced. Carnitine, usually in the form of L-carnitine, is one of the most studied and effective supplements for treating persistent fatigue disorders.[6]

B VITAMINS

The B vitamins are among the most common, and critical, vitamin enzyme cofactors in mammalian physiology, and energy production is no exception. The B vitamins are needed as critical cofactors/coenzymes in many mitochondrial reactions. The B-complex vitamins that act as coenzymes in energy metabolism include thiamin (vitamin B_1), riboflavin (vitamin B_2), niacin, vitamin B_6 (pyridoxine), folate (folic acid), vitamin B_{12} (cobalamin), pantothenic acid, and biotin.[7] Research studies have long suggested that the use of supplements that include B vitamins have positive results with mitochondrial dysfunction.

MAGNESIUM AND MALIC ACID

Magnesium and malic acid play a vital role in the reproduction and function of mitochondria.[8] The mitochondria need magnesium in order to divide in response to energy demands. And ATP, in order to be biologically active, must be bound to a magnesium ion (Mg-ATP). Malic acid is known for its ability to reduce pain and enhance energy, likely due to its role as a Krebs cycle (energy metabolism) intermediate compound.

Supplementing with these key nutrients is a great way to optimize energy, support the mitochondria, relieve FM mimic symptoms, and safeguard your health. Magnesium and malic acid supplementation has been studied and has been shown beneficial in FM. However, it is likely that many of the subjects in these studies actually had mitochondrial dysfunction and not classic FM. The use of magnesium and malic acid may have worked well in these studies mainly by helping to improve energy metabolism and had little direct benefit on mechanisms of classic FM.

Chemical and Food Sensitivities

Chemical and food sensitivities are also believed to play a role in mitochondrial dysfunction. Impaired mitochondrial function may result, in fact, from much lower levels of chemical exposure than many people suppose. It was previously believed that only a heavy dose of toxic chemical exposure would produce a negative health impact, but new scientific research demonstrates that a smorgasbord of low-grade doses can also add up to poor health. Because chemicals are so numerous in our culture, growing numbers of people are developing a wide range of health problems. For example, multiple chemical sensitivity (MCS), which was once nonexistent, is now a concern for many from childhood on. Many minor or major ailments are worsened by the typical daily exposure to these small amounts of many different chemicals delivered to us in products like:

- Air fresheners
- Bleach
- Car exhaust
- Cigarette smoke
- Cosmetics
- Disinfectant
- Fabric softener
- Gas heat
- Herbicides
- Household cleansers

- New carpet and furniture
- Perfume
- Pesticides
- Petroleum products
- Remodeling materials
- Scented laundry soap
- Shampoo
- Toothpaste
- Treated fabric
- Wood smoke

MCS can result from the negative effects of many toxins on critical enzyme pathways. This in turn affects numerous processes in many systems of the body. MCS almost always affects the central nervous system. Symptoms of MCS include—but are far from limited to—depression, fatigue, muscle pain, disorientation, confusion, excessive drowsiness, constipation, diarrhea, and hypothyroidism. You can readily see why MCS might easily be mistaken for FM! This is why assessment of toxic body burden, as well as how well a person can detoxify, is important in the management of chronic health problems, including in those who may have been diagnosed, properly or not, with FM.[9]

Strategies to rid the body of excessive toxins by supporting its detoxifying biochemistry are often a foundational element on the road to recovery, which is why they are a big part of the 21-day Fibro-Fix Foundational Plan.

Reactions to Medication

Medications can also cause functional and metabolic issues, and they are another major cause of mitochondrial damage. In fact, the side effects that so many people experience from drugs may be because they damage the mitochondria.[10] Many classes of drugs are known to adversely affect mitochondria, including:

- Actos/Avandia (medications used in type 2 diabetes)

- Amiodarone (a drug used only in treating life-threatening heart-rhythm disorders)

- Analgesics (acetaminophen)

- Anesthetics, muscle relaxants

- Antibiotics (many)—after all, the mitochondria resemble bacteria in structure and function!

- Anticonvulsants

- Barbiturates

- Beta blockers (class of drugs used in treating heart arrhythmias, protecting the heart from a second heart attack after a first one, and lowering blood pressure)

- Biguanides (like metformin, a drug for prediabetes and type 2 diabetes)

- Chemotherapeutics (some)—cancer medications

- Corticosteroids

- Fibrates

- Neuroleptics (some)—antipsychotic psychiatric medications primarily used to manage psychosis, in particular in schizophrenia and bipolar disorder

- Nucleoside reverse transcriptase inhibitors (antiviral drugs used to treat HIV/AIDS)

- Propofol (a drug used for sedation and the maintenance of general anesthesia)

- Psychotropic drugs

- Statins

This list is not intended to suggest that drugs in these categories should never be used. It's simply to help create awareness that one, or many, of the medications a person is taking may be responsible, at least in part, for some of the FM-like symptoms they are experiencing. Knowledge is power, and understanding this possibility can provide an opportunity for people to work with their prescribing physician to determine if there's a link between the medication and chronic symptoms, so the amount of medications, and doses, can be lowered as much as possible. There are also often alternate medications, as well as nonmedication solutions, to the management of many health issues. Just because the orthodox medical system in Western industrialized countries relies on synthetic drugs almost exclusively to treat people's problems does not mean these are the only possible solutions.

The Functional Fix Plan

The goal when treating functional pain and fatigue syndromes is to redress all contributing imbalances to help the body restore function. Meeting this goal usually requires more than one form of treatment.

Many functional issues require only simple lifestyle changes, such as following the Fibro-Fix Foundational Plan. But I will also recommend supplements in this chapter for specific areas of imbalance. These include supplements for gut repair and for mitochondrial, adrenal, and metabolic support. If the cause of your problem is low thyroid, for instance, with treatment, you can feel better within a few weeks. Other kinds of functional problems can take a little more time to resolve.

SUPPLEMENTS FOR ENHANCING GASTROINTESTINAL HEALTH

- Fiber, 5 to 10 grams of a soluble and insoluble fiber blend

- L-glutamine, 1,500 milligrams per day

- Probiotics, a quality live-culture mixture of beneficial organisms (for example, *Lactobacillus acidophilus, Bifidobacterium longum, Lactobacillus rhamnosus, Lactobacillus casei, Bifidobacterium bifidum, Bifidobacterium breve,* etc.)

- *Saccharomyces boulardii*, a special strain of brewer's yeast that has been extensively studied for its ability to prevent and treat antibiotic-associated diarrheas and *Clostridium difficile*–related diarrhea and to promote optimal gastrointestinal health in general

To conveniently find supplements for this purpose, including the GI-Fix packet and GI-Fix powder, please visit FibroFix.com or DrDavidBrady.com.

SUPPLEMENTS TO SUPPORT CELLULAR ENERGY PRODUCTION

- B-complex vitamins, 50 to 100 milligrams twice daily

- CoQ10, 100 milligrams twice daily

- L-carnitine, 200 to 500 milligrams two or three times daily

- Magnesium, 500 to 1,000 milligrams per day in divided dosages (glycinate or malate form preferred)

- Malic acid, 1,200 to 2,400 milligrams per day in divided dosages

- Mito-Fix and Mito-Fix PQQ*

WHY DO WE NEED PQQ?

Pyrroloquinoline quinone (PQQ) is a water-soluble, vitamin-like compound. While the body can't make PQQ, it can be found in a variety of foods, including parsley, green tea, green peppers, kiwifruit, and papaya. PQQ acts as an antioxidant, encourages the creation of mitochondria, and also protects the nervous system and heart. It may be beneficial in a wide range of conditions associated with mitochondrial dysfunction.

---

* Mito-Fix is a formulary blend of nutrients, nutraceuticals, botanicals, and Krebs cycle intermediates that supports mitochondrial metabolism and energy (ATP) production. Mito-Fix PQQ contains herbs and vitamin-like compounds that support the formation of new mitochondria and increase their density.

To conveniently order supplements for this purpose, check out the Fibro-Fix Metabolic Energy packets or the individual products Mito-Fix and Mito-Fix PQQ capsules at FibroFix.com or DrDavidBrady.com.

EXERCISE AND RELAXATION

Refer to the exercises in Chapter 2 (page 46) and Chapter 5 (page 123) and to the lifestyle recommendations in Chapter 8 (page 221).

Conclusion

In summary, some people who receive an inappropriate diagnosis of FM do not display the entire spectrum of clinical elements indicative of classic FM, and they do not have lab findings that show known pathology or disease. Yet these people do have significant functional problems in their metabolism and possibly in certain organ systems. The functional medicine approach to treatment in such cases is not based on any one specific treatment or solution. It's based on restoring proper cellular biochemistry and metabolism by balancing the hormonal system, correcting nutritional deficiencies, reducing cumulative toxic load and oxidative stress, and optimizing the gastrointestinal environment, among other things. These measures will allow for normal mitochondrial function and cellular energy production and will ultimately lead to a reduction in the signs and symptoms of low energy, fatigue, and often widespread achiness. Doctors sometimes refer to this as a "systems biology" approach, meaning it takes into account many critical and converging processes and biochemical pathways in the body that have to work efficiently for you to feel healthy and vibrant. Testing is done to evaluate these processes (not just the presence or absence of disease) to try to determine where suboptimal function may be occurring so that the identified dysfunctions can be corrected or optimized using the least toxic and most noninvasive methods possible.

Many of these factors can be addressed with simple lifestyle changes, including eating a varied and balanced fresh-food diet (excluding foods that your immune system doesn't tolerate well); consuming targeted vitamin, mineral, and herbal supplements; and managing stress through regular light mobilization and stretching, proper sleep hygiene, adequate recreation, and relaxation techniques (for example, deep-breathing exercises, guided imagery, yoga, meditation, prayer, biofeedback, and other forms of cognitive behavioral therapy).

The old adage that "diagnosis is half the cure" is certainly true. But very targeted and individualized treatment intervention is also key. Therefore, it's always best to work with a health-care practitioner who is well informed about FM, including the disorders often misdiagnosed as FM, and who is also skilled in the functional-medicine approach. A national functional-medicine practitioner search tool can be found on the Web site of the Institute for Functional Medicine at FunctionalMedicine.org to assist you in identifying providers of this type near you. In the next chapter, I will also discuss the best way to bring the knowledge you are acquiring in this book to your doctor.

The last two chapters have shown you how musculoskeletal and functional issues can appear to be fibromyalgia, how you can determine if that is the situation you are in, and what to do when it's not.

But suppose you do not have classic fibromyalgia and your symptoms do not fit into these other two buckets (musculoskeletal and functional)? In the next chapter, I will look at other root causes for chronic pain and fatigue and point you and your physician toward the use of the right diagnostic workups and lab tests to determine what issues may really be causing the problem.

CHAPTER 7

MEDICAL PROBLEMS COMMONLY CONFUSED WITH CLASSIC FM

I f you feel that none of the three buckets described your situation after reading the previous chapters—in other words, if you feel you do not have classic fibromyalgia or a musculoskeletal or functional condition—then there may be some other root cause for your condition that has to be investigated. In this chapter, I will discuss some of the other illnesses that are commonly misdiagnosed as FM. For these types of situations, most of the investigations will require you to work with a physician.

I will point you and your health-care provider toward the right lab tests so that both of you can confirm any conclusions about your condition. While there's no definitive test you can use to diagnose FM, testing can be used to pinpoint the real causes of your problem. Your physician can order these tests. In case your physician is unfamiliar with them, I will provide useful information you can bring to your appointment.

If you decide to bring some of this information to your doctor or other health-care provider, please understand that while some providers maintain an open mind and appreciate the opportunity to learn something new, others may get a little bent out of shape. Just be sure to offer the information with a positive and collaborative tone and spirit, always opening the conversation with how grateful you feel for

FIGURE 7.1 CLINICAL REASONING GUIDE FOR WORKING UP A PATIENT WHO THINKS SHE MAY HAVE FIBROMYALGIA

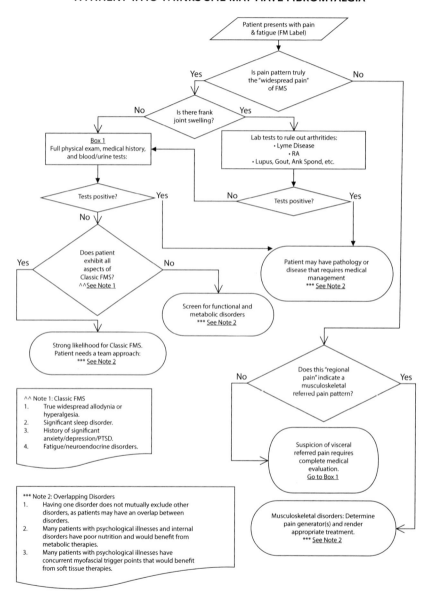

Source: M. J. Schneider, D. M. Brady, and S. M. Perle, "Differential Diagnosis of Fibromyalgia Syndrome: Proposal of a Model and Algorithm for Patients Presenting with the Primary Symptoms of Widespread Pain," Journal of Manipulative and Physiological Therapeutics 29 (2006): 493–501. (Available online at jmptonline.org/issues.)

what your provider has done to assist you. Stress that you are simply sharing some information you have come across in your effort to help yourself. Ask your provider to please look it over. If the answer is no, then you may want to consider looking for another provider. Your current health-care provider may lack the training or perspective to fully understand this approach. If you feel that you do need to find a new provider, or simply add one to your health-care team, I will tell you how to find knowledgeable and open-minded practitioners trained in the functional and integrative medicine approach in the Additional Resources section at the end of this book (page 259).

I am a great believer in the value of lab tests to confirm clinical observations or hypotheses (see Figure 7.1). I'm not talking about testing for the sake of piling up big bills. I'm talking about knowing which tests could alter and refine my decision-making, confirm a diagnosis, and help me to personalize a treatment plan. A treatment plan is based on examining and talking with patients, and then, when these targeted lab tests come back, acting on the data to correct the problem at its core. This is why when people ask me what I do, I tell them I am essentially a medical detective. I dig deep, with applied clinical biochemistry as my tool, in order get to the bottom of what is really wrong, rather than being satisfied with just masking the symptoms.

Basic Screening Tests

As simple as screening tests are to perform, many doctors fail to have any lab tests done on their patients before rendering a FM diagnosis. This is despite the clear guidelines of the American College of Rheumatology that a diagnosis of FM should *never* be rendered until all lab tests come back negative and after no other obvious medical reason for the symptoms has been detected. Your doctor should employ a simple, rational approach to laboratory assessment. Some of the most common tests used are:

- A complete red and white blood cell count (known as a CBC) to help detect anemia, infection, and various blood-based disorders

- C-reactive protein (CRP) and/or erythrocyte sedimentation rate (ESR) to determine if there's significant inflammation in the body

- Thyroid function tests (total and free T3 and T4, TSH, and thyroid antibodies) to screen for overt and functional thyroid disorders

- Standard blood chemistry panel to rule out significant disease or dysfunction of major organs and systems

- Lyme testing (using the Western blot test as a minimum rather than the more common ELISA screening test; more advanced Lyme tests, discussed later in this chapter, are often used if the history and clinical symptoms point to Lyme disease) and, if there seems to be significant joint pain and inflammation, a rheumatic profile to look for autoimmune disorders of the joints

Let's take a closer look at what these tests measure and what they reveal.

Complete Blood Count

A complete blood count (CBC) screens for common forms of anemia (unhealthy or low levels of oxygen-carrying red blood cells sometimes associated with iron and/or B-vitamin deficiencies). It is also used to assess your white blood cells to rule out infection or bone marrow disease.

C-Reactive Protein and/or Erythrocyte Sedimentation Rate

C-reactive protein (CRP) and/or erythrocyte sedimentation rate (ESR) testing can help to confirm the presence or absence of significant levels of inflammation in the body. The CRP test measures levels of C-reactive protein, which will be higher when there's inflammation. The ESR measures how quickly red blood cells sediment—that is, how fast they settle to the bottom of a tube of whole blood. When inflammation is present, red blood cells are denser and settle more quickly. Although the ESR and CRP tests are nonspecific for particular disorders, extremely high values should be followed by further testing to determine if there's an underlying autoimmune disease—such as rheumatoid arthritis, lupus, or multiple sclerosis—or possibly some other undiagnosed serious illness or malignancy.

Thyroid Function Tests

Doctors should routinely perform thyroid blood tests in patients who complain of widespread pain and fatigue in order to rule out obvious hypothyroidism. Most doctors do routinely consider the classic signs and symptoms of low thyroid function, including fatigue, weakness, cold intolerance, low body temperature, weight changes (usually weight gain), and depression. However, common musculoskeletal symptoms of hypothyroidism, such as muscle pain, stiffness, muscle cramping, muscle weakness, numbness and tingling, and joint pain are often overlooked.[1] Yet the incidence of muscle and joint symptoms with hypothyroidism has been reported to be as high as 30 to 80 percent, depending on which study you refer to.

This is extremely important, since it's precisely these vague muscle or joint symptoms that may have driven you to your doctor initially. Like many people, you may be suffering from these or other symptoms, along with fatigue, but are unaware that you have a thyroid condition. If your physician fails to test your thyroid function, it's more likely that your symptoms will inadvertently be misdiagnosed as FM. (For more information on thyroid conditions often missed by standard practitioners, please refer to page 159 of the previous chapter.)

As you have already seen, low thyroid function can produce an inability to think clearly and maintain good cognitive function. And it may also reduce the transit time of food in the gastrointestinal system, which can produce constipation and other symptoms associated with irritable bowel syndrome (IBS) and small intestinal bacterial overgrowth (SIBO).

Fuzzy thinking—as well as all of the symptoms of IBS and SIBO—are also associated with classic FM and can increase the chances of a false diagnosis of FM.

Standard Blood Chemistry Panel

Your doctor should also order a standard blood chemistry panel, a very useful test for evaluating your overall health if you have widespread pain and fatigue. This panel, generally done after an 8 to 10 hour fast, should look at serum blood sugar, glycosylated hemoglobin (HbA1c), liver enzymes (liver function tests, or LFTs), cholesterol and other blood lipids (fats), kidney function, iron, ferritin, and magnesium. Of course, these laboratory tests should be correlated with your medical history, physical examination findings, and other diagnostic tests that your doctor performs. If the physical exam findings suggest that you may be suffering from joint pain or obvious soft tissue inflammation, and not simply increased pain *perception* in the soft tissues, additional laboratory studies—such as a rheumatoid panel, including rheumatoid factor (RF), and antinuclear antibody (ANA), anticyclic citrullinated peptide (ACCP), and uric acid (UA) tests—should be performed, as well.

Lyme Testing

If joint pain, inflammation, and especially neurological symptoms are present, I highly recommend screening for Lyme disease and other tick-borne illnesses. The standard Lyme test using ELISA is notoriously inaccurate and often results in false negatives—and sometimes even false positives. The Western blot test is better but also far from perfect. If the Western blot tests, with their multiple bands, are negative but suspicion of Lyme or other tick-borne illness remains, I often resort to more advanced testing that looks for the DNA/genes of the organisms that cause these infections. I also sometimes use an additional test (known as the iSpot Lyme test) that looks for specific patterns of change in the immune-modulating chemicals known as cytokines, which commonly occur in Lyme and other tick-related infections. To learn more about these advanced Lyme and tick-borne illness tests, which you may want to share with your doctor, visit igenex.com and ispotlyme.com.

Illnesses Testing Can Confirm or Rule Out

If you do not fit any of the buckets discussed in Chapters 4, 5, and 6, then I recommend your doctor investigate whether you may have one of the following:

- Anemia
- Ankylosing spondylitis
- Arachnoiditis
- Cancer
- Lupus
- Lyme disease
- Multiple sclerosis

- Obvious hypothyroidism
- Blood sugar problems
- Rheumatoid arthritis
- Scleroderma
- Small fiber neuropathy
- Stealth infections

Anemia

Anemia results from a lower-than-normal number of or very poor quality red blood cells or low hemoglobin. People with anemia may feel tired and fatigue easily. They may also appear pale, develop palpitations, or become short of breath. Children with anemia are more prone to infections and learning issues.

The main causes of anemia are hemolysis (destruction of red blood cells at too high a rate), bleeding, underproduction of red blood cells (as in a B-vitamin deficiency or bone marrow diseases), and underproduction of hemoglobin (as in sickle cell anemia and iron deficiency anemia). Women are more likely than men to have anemia and iron deficiency because of their menstrual blood loss. Anemia can also come about through gastrointestinal bleeding caused by ulcers, gastritis, or from medications, including such common drugs as aspirin and ibuprofen.

Why is diagnosing anemia important? Because anemia reduces the blood's capacity to carry oxygen to your cells, including your muscles' cells, which use a lot of oxygen. Not only can a lack of oxygen cause poor energy production and fatigue, but it can also force the muscle cells to make energy *without* using oxygen—the anaerobic pathway—and this produces acidic waste products that can accumulate and cause pain or achiness in the muscles. This alternate form of energy production can affect the functioning of the brain, as well, which also requires lots of energy. So you can see how something as simple as undetected and untreated anemia can ultimately result in fatigue, muscle ache, and difficulty with mental sharpness, which can lead to an improper diagnosis of FM.[2]

Ankylosing Spondylitis

Ankylosing spondylitis is an inflammatory disease that can cause some of the vertebrae in your spine and the joints in your pelvis to fuse. The most commonly affected areas are the hip and shoulder joints, lower-back vertebrae, places where tendons and ligaments attach to bones (mainly in the spine, pelvis, and sometimes along the back of the heel), and the cartilage between the breastbone and ribs. Ankylosing spondylitis makes the spine and pelvis less flexible and can affect posture and the ability to move freely. If the ribs are also affected, it may be difficult to take deep breaths. Inflammation can occur in other parts of your body, as well—most commonly, your eyes. This disease typically affects men more than women. Early signs and symptoms may include pain and stiffness in your lower back and hips, especially in the morning and after periods of inactivity. In addition to looking for signs of inflammation in the lab testing, such as the ESR and CRP tests, there are other blood tests that look for genetic predisposition to the disease, including the HLA-B27 test. However, it's often imaging studies, such as x-rays, that ultimately confirm the diagnosis.

Arachnoiditis

Arachnoiditis is inflammation of the arachnoid membranes (thin connective-tissue coverings) surrounding the nerves of the spinal cord. This rare condition can produce a multitude of symptoms, including pain of various types (for example, an intense stinging pain), the feeling that insects are crawling on the skin, tingling, numbness, weakness, muscle cramps, twitching and spasms, bowel and bladder dysfunction, and lower extremity paralysis.

The causes of arachnoiditis include infections from various bacteria or viruses, injury, adhesions or scar tissue, complications from surgery, and other inflammatory processes. Toxic chemicals—including some of the dyes once used in diagnostic medical tests such as myelograms and chemicals found in certain steroid injections, may also give rise to arachnoiditis.

This condition can be very difficult to diagnose. CAT scans, MRIs, and EMG studies are often needed. Arachnoiditis is generally treated with pain medications, and steroid injections and electrical stimulation are sometimes used. But further studies are needed to fully determine whether those treatments are effective. In general, arachnoiditis can produce significant body-wide pain, but it does not generally result in the fatigue, depression, anxiety, and gastrointestinal symptoms that are present in classic FM. This fact should be used by the doctor to help differentiate the two conditions.

Cancer

Cancer begins when cells in some part of the body start to grow abnormally and at a faster-than-usual rate because of damage to DNA. Cancer cells can also travel to other parts of the body in a process called metastasis. What defines a cell as cancerous is that it's growing out of control and invading other tissues. In most but not all cases, cancer cells form a tumor.

When the DNA of a normal cell becomes damaged, the cell either repairs the damage or dies (more accurately it commits suicide in a process known as apoptosis). In a cancer cell, the damaged DNA isn't repaired, and the cell goes on to make new cells, all with the damaged DNA. Sometimes the damage to the DNA is due to a very clear cause, like smoking or some other toxin. At other times, no clear cause can be found. What we do know is that cancer rates have continued to rise with the number of toxins we are exposed to in modern life—in our food, water, and air and in products and drugs we are exposed to that contain harmful chemicals. With cancer, numerous abnormalities usually appear on a comprehensive blood chemistry, indicative of the damage and dysfunction of the organs and systems being affected by the disease. Doctors are trained to be alert to these danger signs.[3]

Lupus

Lupus is a chronic autoimmune disease that occurs when the body's immune system attacks its own tissues and organs. Inflammation caused by lupus can affect the joints, skin, kidneys, blood cells, brain, heart, and lungs. Some people may be born with a tendency toward lupus, which may be triggered by infections, certain drugs, or perhaps even sunlight.[4]

Lupus can be difficult to diagnose because its signs and symptoms often mimic those of other ailments. The most distinctive sign of lupus, occurring in most cases, is a facial rash that resembles the wings of a butterfly across the nose and cheeks. Lab tests such as the antinuclear antibody test, while not definitive or specific for lupus, are highly suggestive of it and should be promptly correlated with other clinical symptoms and imaging studies of the affected tissues and organs.

Signs and symptoms may come on suddenly or develop slowly, and they may be mild or severe, temporary or permanent. Most people have "flares"—when signs and symptoms get worse—and then their symptoms improve or even disappear completely for some time. The most common signs and symptoms are:

- Butterfly-shaped facial rash

- Chest pain

- Dry eyes

- Fatigue and fever

- Fingers and toes turning white or blue when exposed to cold or stress (Raynaud's phenomenon)

- Headaches, confusion, and memory loss

- Joint pain, stiffness, and swelling

- Shortness of breath

- Skin lesions that worsen with sun exposure

Lyme Disease

Lyme is an infectious disease caused by bacteria transmitted by ticks. Early symptoms may include fever, headache, and fatigue. If untreated, symptoms may include joint pain, severe headaches with neck stiffness, heart palpitations, and loss of mobility in the face. Some individuals develop shooting pains or tingling in their arms and legs as well as various other neurological problems. About 10 to 20 percent of people also have memory problems.

Usually, a tick must be attached to the body for 36 to 48 hours before the bacteria can spread. The disease is not believed to be transmissible between people, by other animals, or through food.

Prevention includes efforts to prevent tick bites, such as wearing long pants. Ticks can be removed using tweezers. If the tick is engorged with blood, the antibiotic doxycycline may be used prophylactically to prevent development of infection. I generally recommend this since even though development of this infection is rare, it can be devastating if it does develop, and it becomes very hard to deal with if not treated soon after becoming infected. In acute or new infections, an immediate course of antibiotics—generally, doxycycline, amoxicillin, or cefuroxime—is usually effective. Some people develop a fever and muscle and joint pains from treatment, which may last 1 or 2 days.

Lyme disease is estimated to affect 300,000 people a year in the United States and 65,000 people a year in Europe, but many physicians and experts believe the numbers are actually much higher and growing at epidemic proportions.

Multiple Sclerosis

Multiple sclerosis (MS) is an autoimmune disorder of the nervous system. As with FM, there's a strong female dominance in the disorder, as women are twice as likely as men to be diagnosed with MS. Most people are diagnosed between the ages of 15 and 60, and there's a slightly higher risk of developing MS if the person also has other autoimmune disorders, such as auoimmune thyroid disease, type 1 diabetes, or inflammatory bowel disease.[5]

In MS, the body's immune system attacks and eventually destroys the protective myelin coating or sheath that surrounds the nerves throughout the body, including within the central nervous system, ultimately interfering with the transmission of nerve electrical signals between the brain, spinal cord, and the rest of the body. This can result in a myriad of symptoms, including numbness, tingling, pain, muscle weakness, spasm, twitching, balance and walking problems, fatigue, constipation, diarrhea, excessive urge to urinate, urinary and bowel incontinence, depression, trouble speaking or swallowing, blurred vision, and other eye problems, among others.[6] With this symptom list, it's not hard to imagine how, especially in the early stages, MS can sometimes be confused with FM.

There is no one universally known cause for MS, but various environmental triggers have been associated with the disorder, including viruses; gut bacteria; heavy metals, like mercury and lead; other toxic chemicals; and even vitamin D deficiency.[7] As with most autoimmune disorders, MS is thought to result from a combination of genetic susceptibility combined with exposure—and overreaction—to an environmental trigger. This causes the immune system to attack body tissues with structural characteristics similar to those of the offending environmental trigger (this is often referred to as molecular mimicry).

Generally, an accurate diagnosis can eventually be made using neurological testing, including CAT scans, and even chemical analysis of the cerebrospinal fluid by way of a spinal tap. Conventional treatment for MS generally revolves around reducing the excessive immune response with strong medications known as biologics, which can be very effective in managing or controlling symptoms but carry a risk of serious side effects, including life-threatening infections and elevated cancer risk, especially for blood-based cancers, like lymphoma and leukemia. In functional medicine, the treatment emphasis with MS, as with any autoimmune disease, is on:

- Positively altering the terrain (that is, the overall physiological environment) of the individual and helping quiet the immune system by testing for known triggers and eliminating them[8]

- Optimizing intestinal balance and function (by addressing any dysbiosis and leaky gut using tools like the GI-MAP stool analysis)[9]

- Testing for foods that trigger an immune response (for example, using the ALCAT test) and eliminating them from the diet[10]

- Assuring vitamin D sufficiency

- Testing for and eliminating heavy-metal toxic burden[11]

- Liberal use of omega-3 fatty acids from concentrated fish oil[12]

- Consuming an anti-inflammatory and whole-food organic diet with a supportive supplement program

Obvious Hypothyroidism

Hypothyroidism is discussed at length in Chapter 6 (page 159).

Blood Sugar Problems

A very common medical condition that can lead to a misdiagnosis of FM is problem with blood sugar levels. Although unlikely to cause pain and achiness, blood sugar issues can cause other symptoms associated with FM, such as fatigue, weakness, and cognitive difficulties. If you happen to have musculoskeletal problems, as well, such as myofascial pain syndrome, muscle spasm due to stress or repetitive strain, or postural distortions, you may also experience muscle pain. This can create a common scenario—where multiple problems cause the patient and the doctor to interpret all those symptoms as one condition. This sets the table for an inappropriate FM diagnosis.

While very serious blood sugar problems are linked to diabetes, many people who do not have actual diabetes still have poor blood sugar regulation. This may be due to a poor diet or to insulin resistance or insensitivity often associated with overweight or obesity. In the condition known as reactive hypoglycemia, blood sugar levels fall too low, usually after an excessive output of insulin following a sugary or heavy carbohydrate meal. This drop causes the person to then crave *more* sugar, thus repeating the cycle over and over.

Elevated glucose or elevated glycosylated hemoglobin (HbA1c) on an initial fasting blood chemistry panel may be a clue that you are on that cycle. But just as often, this is not the case. Another approach I use is to order a fasting glucose and insulin level test, then have the person consume a specific amount of sugar, and then retest the glucose and insulin levels at 30-minute intervals for up to 4 hours. This helps to detect blood sugar control abnormalities by looking at how the body reacts to that sugar over a period of time. Once found, these abnormalities can generally be addressed with better dietary choices, including fewer simple carbohydrates, more lean protein with each meal, and nutrient-rich supplements, including a quality multivitamin, chromium, alpha-lipoic acid, and the herbs cinnamon and berberine, all of which can aid in sugar control. In some cases, blood sugar control abnormalities may require the use of medications, such as metformin (Glucophage).

Rheumatoid Arthritis

Rheumatoid arthritis (RA) is a chronic inflammatory disorder that affects the lining of the small joints in the hands and feet, causing painful swelling that can result in bone erosion and joint deformity. RA is an autoimmune disorder, in which your immune system attacks your body's own tissues. In addition to affecting the joints, RA can also sometimes affect the skin, eyes, lungs, and blood vessels.

Although rheumatoid arthritis can occur at any age, it usually begins after age 40 and is much more common among women than men. Symptoms include tender, swollen joints, stiffness, nodules under the skin on the arms, fatigue, fever, and weight loss.

An antibody called the rheumatoid factor (RF), which can be detected by a simple blood test, can be found in the blood of 80 percent of people with rheumatoid arthritis. Possible risk factors for developing rheumatoid arthritis include genetic background, smoking, silica inhalation, periodontal disease, and overgrowth of specific opportunistic microbes present in the gut and/or urinary tract (for example, *Klebsiella, Citrobacter,* and *Proteus*).[13] Conventional treatment involves a combination of patient education, rest and exercise, dietary changes, joint protection, medications, and occasionally surgery. Medications used in the conventional treatment of rheumatoid arthritis include NSAIDs, DMARDs (disease-modifying antirheumatic drugs), TNF-alpha inhibitors, IL-6 inhibitors, T-cell activation inhibitors, B-cell depletors, JAK inhibitors, immunosuppressants, and steroids. While many of these medications are required, based on the severity of the disease and level of patient disability and discomfort, they also carry risks of serious side effects, including gastritis, duodenitis, ulcers, liver and kidney damage, life-threatening infections, and elevated cancer risk, especially for blood-based cancers, like lymphoma and leukemia. In functional medicine, the treatment emphasis with RA, as any autoimmune disease, is on:

- Positively altering the terrain (that is, the overall physiological environment) of the person and helping quiet the immune system by testing for known triggers and eliminating them

- Optimizing intestinal balance and function (by addressing any dysbiosis and leaky gut using tools like the GI-MAP stool analysis)

- Testing for foods that trigger an immune response (for example, using the ALCAT test) and eliminating them from the diet

- Assuring vitamin D sufficiency

- Testing for and eliminating heavy-metal toxic burden

- Liberal use of omega-3 fatty acids from concentrated fish oil

- Consuming an anti-inflammatory and whole-food organic diet with a supportive supplement program

Scleroderma

Scleroderma (pronounced skleer-oh-DUR-muh) is a group of rare diseases that involve the hardening and tightening of the skin and connective tissues, such as collagen—the fibers that provide the framework and support for the body.

In some people, scleroderma affects only the skin. But in many people, scleroderma also harms structures beyond the skin—such as blood vessels, internal organs, and the digestive tract. Signs and symptoms vary, depending on which structures are affected.

Scleroderma affects women more often than men and most commonly occurs between the ages of 30 and 50. While there's no cure for scleroderma, a variety of treatments can ease symptoms and improve quality of life. Here are some signs of this condition.

- **Skin**—Nearly everyone who has scleroderma experiences a hardening and tightening of patches of skin. These patches may be shaped like ovals or straight lines. The number, location, and size of the patches vary by the type of scleroderma. Skin can appear shiny because it's so tight, and movement of the affected area may be restricted.

- **Fingers or toes**—One of the earliest signs of scleroderma is an exaggerated response to cold temperatures (along with emotional distress), which can cause numbness, pain, or color changes (usually blue or purple) in the fingers or toes. Called Raynaud's phenomenon, this condition also occurs in people who don't have scleroderma.

- **Digestive system**—In addition to acid reflux, which can damage the section of esophagus nearest the stomach, some people with scleroderma may also have problems absorbing nutrients if their intestinal muscles aren't moving food properly through the intestines (a process known as peristalsis).

- **Heart, lungs, or kidneys**—Rarely, scleroderma can affect the function of the heart, lungs, or kidneys. These problems can become life-threatening.

Scleroderma is generally conventionally treated, like most inflammatory and autoimmune disorders, with strong anti-inflammatory and immune-suppressing medications that have long and serious side-effect profiles. These may be necessary to halt progressive organ damage but should be limited as much as possible and augmented with the functional medicine approach discussed previously in this chapter for other autoimmune disorders.

Small Fiber Neuropathy

Small fiber neuropathy is not a rare disorder; in fact, it affects up to 40 million Americans. Accurately diagnosing it can be challenging, though, since it manifests as a variety of symptoms. These may include burning or shooting pain, hypersensitivity to pain (hyperalgesia), and interpretation of things that should not be painful, such as light touch, as painful (allodynia)—hence its potential to mimic FM.[14] As with most disorders, an initial diagnosis of small fiber neuropathy is generally determined by a health-care provider doing a comprehensive history and physical exam. However, functional neurophysiologic testing and evaluation of nerve fiber density in the skin (intraepidermal), usually performed by a neurologist, are necessary to provide an accurate diagnosis.

One clue to the presence of small fiber neuropathy is true full-body hyperalgesia, or even allodynia, without the presence of other common characteristics of classic FM, such as depression, anxiety, IBS, and history of trauma or abuse. The proper management of small fiber neuropathy will depend on the underlying reason for its development. Treatments include antidepressants, anticonvulsants, opioid medications, topical pain-relieving therapies (lidocaine), and some nonpharmacologic treatments used for various forms of neuropathic pain, such as cool or warm soaks, soft socks, and foot tents. Transcutaneous electrical nerve stimulation, acupuncture, physical therapy, and massage have also been used, but these treatments have not been examined in clinical trials for small fiber neuropathic pain.

Stealth Infections

A common problem, which often goes undetected by conventional medical diagnosis, is the presence of ongoing chronic stealth infections—meaning subtle and hidden infections. Viruses can cause ongoing fatigue, lethargy, muscle ache, and immune suppression without causing an acute or readily identifiable infection, as with a cold or flu.[15] Viruses like Epstein-Barr virus, which in the acute form causes mononucleosis ("mono"), stay in the body forever once you are exposed to

SCREENING FOR PERSISTENT VIRAL INFECTIONS

I frequently screen people who come into my office with long-term achiness and fatigue for common persistent viral infections using antibody titer tests (such as IgG/IgM antibodies and viral capsid antigen) for various common viral organisms (especially Epstein-Barr virus and cytomegalovirus). I also look at the levels and ratios of the various subtypes of white blood cells (leukocytes)—including absolute hymphocytes, CD4, CD8, the CD4/CD8 ratio, and CD57—all of which can give insight into the likely level of viral load and infection.

them. But a healthy immune system will generally keep them in check. However, in some people, particularly those with immune suppression from chronic stress, the immune system cannot adequately control the virus, and it can lurk around causing persistent but lower-level symptoms. In addition to Epstein-Barr virus, some of these viruses include:

- Cytomegalovirus

- Herpes simplex virus

- Hepatitis viruses

- Human T-cell lymphotropic virus family

Persistent stealth viral infections have been implicated in autoimmune diseases and various forms of cancer, but very often they simply cause vague, ongoing fatigue and achiness. Just think about how you feel when you get an acute viral infection, such as a cold or flu. You feel extreme fatigue, and all of your muscles ache. If you had fatigue and achiness all the time from a chronic, lower-level viral infection, can you see how you might be mistakenly diagnosed with FM?

There are numerous treatment options to deal with ongoing low-level viral infections. Various classes of antiviral medications are available, but they often have serious side effects, including liver damage. They can also be quite expensive. Generally, they are more effective in acute infections as opposed to chronic or low-level stealth infections. For chronic infections, I use natural agents that boost the body's natural killer cells (NK-cells) and other immune system functions, as well as agents that act as direct antivirals. These may include:

- High doses of vitamin C (including intravenous infusions)

- Immune-stimulating botanicals (such as elderberry, astragalus, echinacea, and goldenseal)

- Plant-based NK-cell stimulators, including a multitude of active compounds derived from mushrooms, fungi, and other organisms (for example, extracts from the mushrooms cordyceps, shiitake, maitake, and reishi; the active compound beta-1,3 glucan from fungal cell walls; and arabinogalactan from the larch tree)

- Fatty acids such as lauric acid in the form of monolaurin, which can help dissolve the phospholipid sheath, or covering, that stealthy encapsulated viruses cover or cloak themselves with as they leave your body's cells in order to hide from the immune system

For your convenience, some immune-enhancing supplement options and formulations, such as Immuno-Fix, can be found on FibroFix.com and DrDavidBrady.com.

Conclusion

In this chapter, we looked at some of the other root causes—besides classic fibromyalgia and musculoskeletal and functional disorders—that may be causing your condition. You also learned how to explore these other avenues with your doctor, often through further testing, and many specific lab tests to support your investigations were mentioned. You were also encouraged, if necessary, to find a different practitioner, one with a more sophisticated understanding of fibromyalgia and the illnesses that mimic it.

In the next and final chapter, I will present a program for following through and consolidating all the gains you have made so far.

CHAPTER 8

MOVING FORWARD FIBRO-FREE

In this chapter, you'll make your gains permanent by learning how to follow a long-term maintenance program.

To begin with, continue to follow through on all that you have learned in the previous chapters. For instance, if you discovered that your pain was caused by a musculoskeletal problem, it's essential that you continue to follow the program in Chapter 5. You also must continue to get regular adjustments and bodywork and do whatever else your chiropractor or physical therapist recommends to keep you functional and in musculo-skeletal balance.

If you discovered that a metabolic dysfunction was the cause of your pain syndrome, complete the treatment protocol in Chapter 6. In some cases, you may be adding a dietary change, nutritional supplement, botanical/herbal remedy, or prescription medication (for example, support for your thyroid) that you or your physician has identified as appropriate for your condition. This may require retesting at certain intervals, such as semiannually or annually, to assure that your functions are restored. Make sure to do that!

And if you discovered that you do indeed have classic FM, then it's essential that you follow the combination program I recommend in Chapter 4 until you're pain-free and have recaptured your energy and vitality.

No matter what category seems to fit your situation, many of the positive health and lifestyle recommendations made in this book will continue to provide benefits for you. For instance, if you did well with the 21-day Fibro-Fix Foundational Plan, then there's no reason to not reengage in it every 4 to 6 months or to work a quality high-protein, nutrient-dense shake into your daily routine—perhaps by starting your day with it. There are some great smoothie options (see page 234) and offered at FibroFix.com. If you felt better with some of the stress reduction practices, movement exercises, muscle and soft-tissue self-therapy, and other suggestions up to this point in the book, by all means continue to make these a part of your everyday routine.

But if, having read to this point, it seems that your pain and fatigue don't fit the pattern of classic fibromyalgia or the profiles of the other buckets either, then you need to follow the instructions in Chapter 7, and in conjunction with your doctor, get the tests you need to find the root—or roots—of your problem. You aren't ready to follow the maintenance recommendations described in this chapter until you have identified the nature of your pain syndrome and have taken steps to address it. Once you have done so, then secure your recovery by following the recommendations outlined here—which I advise all recovering pain and fatigue sufferers follow, regardless of the cause of their illnesses.

10 Recommendations for Living a Healthy Life

Once you have discovered the root of your pain and fatigue issue and have begun to recover, you'll need to identify the types of changes that will support your new and hard-won health and well-being. The everyday choices you make have a profound effect on your overall health. Which basic principles will contribute to your wellness? Is there some way to boil down the hundreds and thousands of health tips that we are barraged with in magazines, on TV, and from our friends, neighbors, and relatives? The answer is yes. I do it in my practice all the time. Here are my 10 easy-to-follow impactful recommendations that make a difference.[1]

1. Eat a healthy diet.

2. Supplement your diet with critical vitamins and minerals.

3. Exercise and move regularly.

4. Reduce your stress level.

5. Make time for relaxation and sleep.

6. Maintain a sense of purpose and accomplishment.

7. Clean up your environment.

8. Keep it simple!

9. Have fun.

10. Make your health a priority.

1. Eat a Healthy Diet

Almost no topic I can think of is as important, as emotional, and as confusing as diet. The way we eat is personal—driven by our feelings, by our cultural history, by peer pressure and socialization. Your friends or your kids want to go out for pizza? It's hard to say no, but what about the gluten and cheese? It can be hard to stay on the diet that's right for you— and yet perhaps nothing has a greater effect on your overall health and longevity than your diet. No amount of supplements, exercise, or stress management can change that fact.

You may have already realized that until you began to follow the Fibro-Fix Eating Plan, your eating habits weren't the greatest. You've now experienced the benefits of making a positive nutritional change. But how do you carry that forward?

Well, if you look at all the diet books on the shelf, your confusion will probably only deepen since many of those diets contradict one another. Low carb or no carb? Low fat or no fat? High or low protein? Grains or no grains? Which one do you believe? Which one is *right*? In a sense, they may all be right since no diet is right for every person. We're individuals with different bodies, biochemical idiosyncrasies, and preferences. Scientists and physicians call this variation *genetic uniqueness* (though they rarely pay any attention to that when recommending diets or giving health advice). And the government certainly doesn't consider genetic uniqueness when making public dietary guidelines. It's easier to put everyone into one big box.

In my clinical practice, I have seen positive benefits from all kinds of different diets. The trick is to figure out which one fits your situation. That may require a bit of trial and error, but it will be worth the effort if it helps you remain pain-free, feel more energetic, and have greater vitality and mental clarity. Eggs are a nutritious food, but if they trigger an allergic or sensitivity response, then they're no good for you, at least right now. It's also crucial to understand the specific factors that make any diet healthy or unhealthy. Here are some general suggestions that can be applied to any dietary style.

- Eat fresh, unprocessed foods whenever possible.

- Eat lots of fresh vegetables and reasonable amounts of fresh fruit every day.

- Limit your consumption of grain-fed and corn-fed saturated animal fats and hydrogenated trans-fatty acids.

- Eat lean protein with every meal or snack.

- Don't overeat.

- Time eating properly.

- Maintain proper water and fluid consumption.

- Limit alcohol consumption.

Let's look at these in greater depth.

EAT FRESH, UNPROCESSED FOODS WHENEVER POSSIBLE

One of my mentors once said to me, "*The less doctored the foods you eat, the less doctoring you'll need.*" Today this is truer than ever before.[2] Prepackaged convenience foods are full of additives, preservatives, and all sorts of chemicals with unpronounceable names. Keep this in mind while shopping: Shop around the outside edges of most supermarkets. That's where the *real* food is! Though the potential health concerns of genetically modified organisms (GMOs) have yet to be fully understood, the benefits of fresh produce, regardless of possible modification, still far outweigh the concerns when compared to processed, prepackaged foods.

But even fresh produce can have its problems. Often, it's full of toxic pesticide and herbicide residues and molds that can be harmful when consumed. That's why it's best to wash all vegetables and fruit completely. Using a veggie/fruit soak is much better at removing chemicals than water alone. Letting your fruits and veggies soak in a large pot of clean water with a tablespoon of apple cider vinegar or white vinegar for 15 to 30 minutes before thoroughly rinsing them can also do wonders to remove these toxins.

Try to purchase fresh, organic, non-GMO produce if it's available and within your budget. Buying organic may lower your exposure to pesticide toxins and genetically altered products. I also tell my patients to apply a simple test to the meal they are about to eat: Look down at your plate and ask yourself one question: *Could I have purchased this food as is 100 years ago?* If the answer is yes, then you probably bought fresh food.

EAT LOTS OF FRESH VEGETABLES AND REASONABLE AMOUNTS OF FRESH FRUIT EVERY DAY

Liberal consumption of fresh vegetables and moderate amounts of fruits can help reduce cancer, heart disease, and many other health disorders.[3] These fresh whole foods contain protective antioxidant and anticarcinogenic vitamins, minerals, phytonutrients, and fiber. But remember, too, that fruits can be very high in sugar and may be a problem if you have blood sugar issues. For example, grapes contain healthful antioxidants, but they also contain high levels of sugar. Grapes are fine for some but problematic for those with blood sugar problems or weight gain. And if you're trying to consume a moderate carbohydrate diet, be sure that the vegetables you select are fresh, unprocessed, and limited in sugars and starches. When Congress characterized french fries and ketchup as "vegetables," it reinforced the ever-present confusion about which vegetables are healthy and which are best avoided due to their high starch content. Potatoes are just one example of a starchy vegetable. Although a baked potato is healthier than french fries, and far better than chips, the potato's high levels of starchy carbs mean that you should limit your consumption.

Starchy Vegetables to Limit

- Corn
- Parsnips
- Peas

- Potatoes
- Pumpkin
- Yams

LIMIT YOUR CONSUMPTION OF GRAIN-FED AND CORN-FED SATURATED ANIMAL FATS AND HYDROGENATED TRANS-FATTY ACIDS

The excessive consumption of animal fats from meats, eggs (yolks), and dairy has been linked in some studies to the development of cancer and heart disease. This doesn't mean that you should never consume these products, but if you do, eat them in moderation and in the correct forms.

For example, try to eat poultry or fish instead of normal commercial beef or pork the majority of the time. Of particular concern are commercially raised meats. These animals are fed corn and grains rather than their natural diet of grass. And part of the corn—the oil—is converted in the animal's system to a very inflammatory fat called arachidonic acid. When we consume the animal's flesh, the arachidonic acid is incorporated into our cells, causing our bodies to become much more prone to inflammation (pain and swelling) when our tissues are stressed or traumatized. This may at least partially explain why Western industrialized countries, where most commercially fed animals are produced and eaten, have such a high incidence of inflammatory disorders like heart disease, prediabetes, rheumatoid arthritis, lupus, and multiple sclerosis, among others.

Free-range, grass-fed animals, such as buffalo, don't have this problem, and are much healthier to consume. Free-range beef and poultry are also available in more areas now, and although more expensive, are worth the investment. After all, some of the healthiest cultures on the planet have traditionally eaten a great deal of animal fat and protein—but the animals they consume aren't raised on commercial grains; they mature naturally, consuming grass and other foods they were designed to eat.

There has been a massive media campaign over the past several decades aimed at getting people to eat less animal fat. Unfortunately, the products the food industry has developed to replace animal fats are unhealthy and should be avoided. Hydrogenated oils, like margarine, contain trans fats and have been linked to many metabolic problems, and they are far worse than even large amounts of natural saturated fats, including butter.[4] The new nonfat and low-fat food products flooding the marketplace contain a multitude of synthetic oils and other chemicals that can result in deficiencies of essential fats and fat-soluble vitamins, and they have gastrointestinal side effects. The general rule is that if you're going to consume fats, choose the natural versus the synthetic fat. That's right—use butter instead of margarine. But use it in moderation!

EAT LEAN PROTEIN WITH EVERY MEAL OR SNACK

It's very important that you eat lean protein with every meal and snack.[5] Eating the typical bagel, English muffin, or toast alone for breakfast isn't recommended. Consumption of high-carb foods, especially without balancing them with protein, can result in low energy an hour or two after eating (this is known as reactive hypoglycemia, as discussed in Chapter 7) and weight gain. Always consume protein at breakfast to get a good start to your day. I suggest moderate consumption of eggs in the morning. And I strongly encourage you to eat free-range, organic eggs. The feed commercial chickens are given results in egg yolks with more inflammatory fats, such as arachidonic acid, and fewer beneficial fats and nutrients. You don't need to avoid yolks from free-range, organic chickens. Yes, even if you have high cholesterol! Quality protein powders— such as whey (unless you're allergic or sensitive to dairy), pea, and hemp—are also a convenient way to consume protein in the morning, as well as at other times during the day. Many of these protein powders are also fortified with valuable vitamins, minerals, and fibers and can serve as a large part of your nutritional supplement program without having to swallow a lot of pills. Convenient ideas and options for protein shakes can be found on FibroFix.com or DrDavidBrady.com.

DON'T OVEREAT

Overeating puts a strain on your body, especially if you're eating junk food. Burning food to create energy actually requires many vitamins and minerals, so if your food isn't high quality, your body will use up its reserves of these critical nutrients to process the excess calories and to keep your biochemistry running. Junk foods don't contain enough vitamins even to adequately metabolize the food itself! The result? Fatigue and a multitude of health problems.

In addition, many by-products of foods can be toxic, and your body must process and eliminate them. The detoxification of these substances requires many of the same vitamins and minerals you need to burn the food to produce energy. So, overeating depletes vitamin and mineral stores this way, too. And if overeating continues, the excessive toxic load can also put a strain on your liver, kidneys, and other organ systems, as well as on your overall metabolism.

Consuming more calories than you need over a long period of time eventually leads to obesity, a primary risk factor for today's most common

WHAT ABOUT MY MORNING COFFEE?

The caffeine in the coffee many consume with their high-carb breakfast can profoundly alter biorhythms. That's why drinking that morning cuppa Joe is a hard habit to break. Once relieved of that habit, though, people notice an overall improvement in energy throughout the day. In fact, caffeine intake seems to be neutral to these biorhythms only between about 3 p.m. and 5 p.m. (This, by the way, is precisely British tea time.) If you're going to take in caffeine, try doing it for a while in the late afternoon to see what effect it has, but make sure it is not so late that it interferes with your sleep. I've noticed that those who are sensitive to caffeine may have problems getting to sleep if they consume caffeine after 4 or 5 in the afternoon. (For more information on eating to reinforce healthy biorhythms, you should read *The Circadian Prescription: Get in Step with Your Body's Natural Rhythms* by Dr. Sidney MacDonald Baker and Karen Baar.)

However, most people who have actual classic FM—and the hypervigilance, stress, anxiety, and insomnia that accompany it—generally do better avoiding caffeine altogether.

life-shortening diseases (diabetes, high blood pressure, and heart disease, to name just a few). The easiest way to extend life span in animals is to restrict their caloric intake—not enough to starve them, but enough so that they aren't consuming more than necessary. This is also true for humans.[6] We have discussed the mitochondria a lot in this book and how important they are to the production of energy in the cells of the body. Restricting your calories even marginally results in a phenomenon called mitochondrial biogenesis, or the production of more mitochondria in each cell. This translates into more energy and vitality!

Westerners, and most dramatically Americans, eat far more food and calories than is required to live on a daily basis. However, we have become used to this, so our bodies expect it and crave the food when it does not arrive in our stomachs. It takes a while to retrain yourself, but it can be done over a fairly short period, within a couple of weeks. Eat only until your hunger has ceased. It isn't healthy to eat until you feel engorged and "stuffed." Save that for Thanksgiving. Eat less and live better and longer!

TIME YOUR EATING PROPERLY

The standard American three-large-meals per day way of eating isn't the best approach to maintain stable blood sugar and insulin levels. Do you think our early ancestors planned three tightly scheduled meals per day or just ate one huge meal in the evening because they were too busy and stressed during the day to consider eating? Very likely, they ate mainly as they found food. Many nutritionists and physicians suggest that it may be better to eat smaller, more frequent meals—and that our meals contain some protein whenever carbohydrates are consumed. While there is a lack of firm scientific data to prove this hypothesis, and a person with good blood sugar control should be able to tolerate not eating for a considerable amount of time without feeling faint or lethargic, more and more evidence suggests that our eating patterns affect our normal hormonal biorhythms. Our hormones and neurotransmitters have been patterned over hundreds of thousands of years—not to sit down at a table and eat a large prepared meal three times per day but to eat a bit more frequently and during the times of day that were suitable for finding food and prey. Although our ancestors probably rarely, if ever, sat down to a large late-evening meal, we have become accustomed to doing just that in our busy and stress-filled lives.

In terms of when to eat what, clinical trials show that about 50 percent of individuals report feeling better when they eat protein-based foods in the morning and consume most of their carbohydrates in the late afternoon or very early evening.[7] Which happens to be exactly the opposite of the bagel-and-coffee or cereal-and-fruit breakfasts and the high-protein, meat-containing dinners of the standard American diet (SAD). In fact, that's an appropriate acronym for the American diet—sad, because it usually is very SAD indeed.

In summary, many people benefit from eating smaller meals more frequently. This is the so-called grazing approach to eating. However, if the foods selected are high in sugar and starches, it can create destructive blood sugar peaks and valleys due to reactive hypoglycemia, essentially putting you on a blood sugar roller coaster, where you constantly eat and crave sweets. The key is to be careful about the foods you select— to avoid crackers, cookies, bagels, and candy and instead to consume whole foods, such as raw and cooked nonstarchy fresh vegetables, reasonable amounts of relatively low-carbohydrate fruits (such as berries), nuts, eggs, and meats. Basically, this means you should consider the timing of when you eat food as well as paying attention to the rules that preceded this one, such as eating the right kinds of foods, not overeating, and consuming lean protein with each meal or snack.

MAINTAIN PROPER WATER AND FLUID CONSUMPTION

We're made up mostly of water, the magical solvent within which millions and millions of chemical reactions occur in our bodies. We all need to consume adequate amounts of pure water every day—about six 8-ounce glasses per day is generally recommended. But this doesn't include the ice cubes in your scotch on the rocks or the water in your fruity drink, either! Preferably, it should be plain pure water. Use spring water from a trusted source or reverse-osmosis filtered water.

On the other hand, don't drink too much water or other liquids with meals since this dilutes your stomach acid and enzymes and can impair digestion. If you need to drink with meals, drink pure water slightly acidified with the juice of a fresh lemon wedge or two. If you need something a little more interesting, instead of soda or sugary drinks, try a refreshing spritzer made of ice, $^2/_3$ of a glass of sparkling water, and $^1/_3$ fresh fruit juice.

Although more and more people are questioning this assumption, most people expect that when they turn on the tap, their water will be fresh and clean. That is not always so. Tap water from municipal supplies isn't nearly as good as government sources would have you believe. The water from your local municipal treatment facility is now commonly contaminated with a variety of toxic chemicals; heavy metals; and pesti-

THE FIBRO-FIX MAINTENANCE DIET

I recommend that you continue to follow a basic anti-inflammatory, allergen-free diet, along with a basic program of helpful supplements, to assure that you have good nutrition. This diet, the Fibro-Fix Maintenance Diet, is gluten-free, soy-free, and dairy-free and contains adequate protein from either animal or vegetarian sources, as well as lots of phytonutrients from fresh organic fruits and vegetables. It's essential that you consume enough protein with meals and snacks to keep your blood sugar stable throughout the day and to keep your detoxification pathways humming.

To help you create meals of fresh, unprocessed foods going forward, you'll find sample meal plans here and full recipes in the Fibro-Fix Recipes section at the end of this book (page 234). Feel free to get creative using the basic guidelines.

SAMPLE BREAKFAST OPTIONS

3 poached eggs over a bed of fresh spinach
2 to 3 slices of turkey bacon with sliced avocado and tomato
2 to 3 hard-cooked eggs with $^1/_2$ grapefruit
$^2/_3$ cup hot quinoa cereal or gluten-free steel cut oats with 1 scoop protein powder (containing about 8 to 10 grams of protein), $^1/_2$ cup berries, and a small handful of walnuts or pecans

cide, herbicide, antibiotic, and other prescription drug residues.[8] It's also a common practice to remove solid particles during water treatment by mixing aluminum sulfate into the water. Yet, aluminum toxicity has been increasingly linked to disorders such as Alzheimer's disease, Parkinson's disease, and ADHD (attention deficit hyperactivity disorder).[9]

Chlorination and fluoridation are also double-edged swords. While they can kill microbes and help eliminate dental cavities, they also create oxidative stress in your body, which may promote various chronic diseases. Chlorine can also form highly toxic and carcinogenic chemicals called organochlorides. Because of this, I always recommend installing a reverse-osmosis or charcoal water filter in your home—at a minimum on

| Breakfast detox scramble: 2 to 3 eggs scrambled with onion and/or garlic |
| Leftover salmon sautéed with veggies |

SAMPLE LUNCH OPTIONS

| Buffalo burger (gluten-free or no bun) with dill coleslaw and tomato slices |
| Black bean soup and green salad topped with avocados and sprouts |
| Baked cod topped with avocado salsa and steamed artichoke |
| Open roast turkey sandwich on gluten-free toast with mustard and sauerkraut |
| Carrot-ginger soup with salad topped with steamed green beans and avocado |

SAMPLE DINNER OPTIONS

| Wild salmon with garlic beet greens and tossed green salad |
| Roast chicken with kale salad and baked squash |
| Organic vegetable broth with garlic sautéed shrimp and vegetables, served with sesame buckwheat noodles |
| Grilled buffalo burger over grilled portobello mushroom served with baby greens salad |
| Roasted cauliflower, broccoli, and Brussels sprouts served with baked acorn squash and a mixed greens salad |
| Broiled chicken with steamed beets and brown rice |
| Baked cod, sole, or flounder and green beans topped with tomato pesto |

your main kitchen sink faucet and optimally on the main water feed to your residence.

LIMIT ALCOHOL CONSUMPTION

There has been a great deal of contradictory information about the consumption of alcohol over the past several years. Some claim that alcohol should not be consumed at all, while others say a moderate amount may be beneficial. It's universally agreed, though, that drinking a lot of alcohol isn't healthy. It puts stress on the liver that eventually can lead to degeneration and cirrhosis. In some individuals, even moderate amounts of alcohol, three or four drinks per day, can lead to elevated blood liver enzymes—indicators of liver cell destruction. Alcohol is also very dehydrating and takes a toll on the lining of the intestines, potentially leading to ulcers or a "leaky gut." A leaky gut lets a higher than normal amount of the food you eat, and other materials, into the bloodstream. This can ultimately result in food sensitivities, added toxicity, immune activation, and, potentially, autoimmune disease.

And yet, people who live in cultures where it's traditional to consume a small amount of alcohol with meals—like the Mediterranean cultures—don't seem to suffer any ill effects from the practice—and may actually derive some value from it. Red wine contains many antioxidants and phytonutrients, like resveratrol and pterostilbene, which have beneficial effects on the body.[10] It also thins the blood slightly, which means that the blood is somewhat less sticky, making it less likely to stick to the walls of arteries and form the clots that can lead to heart attack, pulmonary embolism, and stroke. The effect is similar to taking a baby aspirin each day. (If you're already on blood-thinning medications, check with your doctor before consuming alcohol.) Alcohol can also help lower the so-called bad cholesterol (LDL) while increasing the good cholesterol (HDL). These phenomena probably account for the lower incidence of heart attacks and strokes in those who drink moderately. And alcohol has also been shown to lower blood pressure and reduce the incidence of respiratory diseases, some cancers, and a variety of other health conditions.[11] In fact, a Harvard study revealed a 21 to 28 percent decrease in death rates from all causes in men who were moderate drinkers versus abstainers.[12] A similar study in China showed a 20 percent reduction. The National Institute on Alcohol Abuse and Alcoholism reported that moderate intake of alcohol lengthened life span by 3 percent among white male drinkers compared to nondrinkers.[13]

In general, enjoying an alcoholic beverage occasionally is fine. If you enjoy wine with your dinner, keep it to one or two glasses and select red over white most of the time. This Russian proverb may have put it best: *Drink a glass of schnapps after your soup and steal a ruble from your doctor.*

2. Supplement Your Diet with Critical Vitamins and Minerals

I've pointed out throughout this book how critical it is to have adequate amounts of vitamins and minerals to support the metabolic reactions taking place in your body. In some cases, much larger amounts—therapeutic doses—of supplements are vital for healing and wellness. Although we call them supplements, the truth is that in today's world they are essential.

The supplements I suggest are included to help your body cope with inflammation and to keep your cellular engines running. Here is a minimal program of supplements that will support overall health, vitality, and cellular energy production.

- B-complex, 50 to 100 milligrams twice daily
- Carnitine, 500 milligrams 2 or 3 times daily
- CoQ10, 100 milligrams twice daily
- Curcumin, 200 milligrams daily
- Fish oil, 1 to 2 grams per day (high EPA-DHA content in triglyceride form preferred)
- Magnesium, 500 to 1,000 milligrams per day in divided dosages (glycinate or malate form preferred)
- Multivitamin/mineral (professional-quality version), use per label instructions

Information on convenient daily maintenance nutritional supplements, such as the Fibro-Fix Daily Wellness packets, which provide a baseline support, can be found at FibroFix.com.

3. Exercise and Move Regularly

We've explored the challenges of getting enough exercise—and the right kind of exercise—if you suffer from global pain and fatigue. As your body heals, you'll want to increase the variety and amount of movement and exercise you do. Include forms of exercise in your daily schedule that gradually increase your flexibility and strength, without resulting in metabolic overexertion—in other words, without overdoing it. Once you're no longer experiencing pain and fatigue, you can enjoy a wider range of exercises. But I recommend that you start slowly and stick with simple things like the movement exercises, starting on page 48, along with walking, while building up and increasing your activities gradually.

There is also a lot you can do outside of a formal exercise program. Our society has changed dramatically over the past several generations, resulting in generally sedentary lifestyles. A typical job now consists of sitting in front of a computer screen and talking on the telephone in a sealed windowless room lit by fluorescent light bulbs (often with carpeting that outgasses toxic chemicals). This is a big departure from the occupations of old, such as farming, manufacturing, and construction jobs. Those jobs had their hazards—and their toxins—but they had the advantage of being more physically demanding and often occurred outdoors. The dangers to health of a sedentary lifestyle have been well documented and publicized. The new phrase "Sitting is the new smoking" is accurate and describes how being sedentary during the day has now replaced smoking as one of the most common health risks. Most significant diseases of our time—including heart disease, diabetes, high blood pressure, obesity, and many others—are much more common in populations that are sedentary.[14]

But even under these conditions, there are ways you can exercise more without having to schedule a class or find time for the gym. For starters, don't use the elevator or escalator. Take the stairs whenever possible. Get some saddlebags for your bike, and use it to do your grocery shopping. You'll be shocked how much a bicycle can carry. Walk to the mailbox instead of driving to it, and to keep your interest, measure how far you've walked each day by attaching a pedometer to your belt.

Of course, joining a local health club or gym is also a good idea, particularly if you live in colder climates, where it's difficult to exercise outdoors in the winter. A one-hour commitment several times a week is all it takes. A full-service health club can usually provide you with a balance of aerobic activities (stationary bike-riding, treadmills, stair-steppers, and elliptical machines) as well as important anaerobic activities, such as light-to-moderate strength training (weight machines and free weights).

I have also found short-burst interval training to be effective for those who don't have a lot of time to exercise. New research has suggested that short bursts of high-intensity activity may have a greater overall effect than 20 to 30 minutes of low-intensity aerobic activity.[15] Using a high-intensity step machine, for instance, is good for this type of time-efficient conditioning. Many classes offered at gyms now feature short-duration, high-intensity training activities; a good trainer can help guide you in finding a routine that incorporates this kind of exercise. However, I want to caution those of you who have determined that you have classic FM, or a functional issue, to go slow and not overexert yourself until you have come further along the path of repairing your stress response and metabolic state. If the activity makes you feel worse, then don't do it!

Unfortunately, many people feel intimidated about joining a gym. They may be embarrassed about their bodies, reluctant to look silly using equipment they are unfamiliar with, or even worried about being hit on by the opposite sex. Those attitudes may be a little out of date, though. Health clubs have come a long way and generally are not just meat markets full of muscle heads. My local gym is full of people of all ages working out and helping each other whenever possible.

Clubs exclusively for women have also become quite popular and afford greater security and privacy. By asking around, talking with representatives from your local health clubs, and doing a little investigating, you can find out which clubs in your area have the kind of environment you're looking for. Remember, don't allow anyone to push you too hard, especially if you're recovering from an illness. Exercise needs to be comfortable and enjoyable so you'll want to continue.

Most clubs also have professional athletic trainers who will demonstrate the equipment and help you develop a program tailored to your needs and fitness level—although the level and consistency of education of exercise trainers is highly variable and not standardized. There are really good ones, and then . . . well, you know. Health club memberships do create an added monthly expense, but the investment is well worth it if you want to make your health a priority. But don't waste money paying for a membership unless you're dedicated to making exercise a part of your daily and weekly schedule and are committed to using your gym or club. Remember, the most expensive health club membership is one that's never used.

4. Reduce Your Stress Level

As you have learned in this book, stress can literally cause pain and undermine your metabolism, and it is a major component of classic FM.[16] It's essential going forward for you to adopt constructive ways to calm stress. The first step is to *notice* when your stress begins to ramp up. Mindfulness practices like meditation can help you do this. Similarly, doing yoga a few times a week or more can increase your physical function and help you manage stress. Whether it's yoga, meditation, progressive muscle relaxation, deep breathing, guided imagery, tai chi, qigong, or a range of other cognitive behavioral therapy options, it's essential to find ways to calm your stress. The stress-relieving and calming supplements I have mentioned throughout this book can also support meaningful stress reduction (see pages 102–106).

It has been known for decades that highly stressed people, the so-called type-A personalities, are more prone to high blood pressure, ulcers, and heart attacks.[17] However, it's becoming more and more apparent that stress contributes to a broader array of health problems and that it affects individuals with just about any type of personality. The stress response is a built-in feature of our nervous system, designed to jump-start the fight-or-flight reaction and help us survive a possible threat (the stressor). But as I've discussed at length, stress can be a negative force if it remains in your body and becomes chronic.

Long ago, our stressors were immediate and acute, like turning a corner in the forest and seeing a hostile animal. We ran, climbed, or fought off the beast, or we didn't live to worry about it. Today, stress is chronic—

in the form of the boss we can't stand, the long commute, our shrinking savings, or those huge issues that make us feel helpless, like the debt ceiling, the economy, or terrorism. These stressors are there every day. We can't run, climb, or fight our way out of them. At least not very easily or quickly. And since we don't get to employ the burst of physical energy—resulting from the adrenaline and the other reactions taking place in fight or flight—that blows off the effect of the stress, we end up internalizing it. The results can be muscle tightness, ulcers, high blood pressure, and other deeper problems, such as irritable bowel syndrome and classic FM. At the same time, it's good to remember that although physical action does drain off the stress, too much exercise can itself become a stress to your body, rather than a stress reliever. The key to healthy exercise is moderation.

As I mentioned earlier, your body's stress response primarily involves the adrenal glands. Chronically overactivated adrenal glands put out higher than normal levels of specific hormones (cortisol and the catecholamines) that, among other things, elevate blood sugar and blood pressure, slow thyroid function, and promote weight gain. And once they are exhausted from too much stress-induced activity, the adrenals can cause extreme fatigue and lead, as we have seen, to a false diagnosis of fibromyalgia. Or the stress and adrenal dysfunction can be a major component of classic FM. Worn-out adrenals can also increase our susceptibility to diabetes, hypertension, and a number of other health problems.

A diet of junk and convenience food, rather than fresh vital food, is itself stressful. But the most common dietary stress put on the adrenal glands is probably caffeine. The reason people feel a jolt from caffeine is the adrenal-gland stimulation it provides—the initiation of the fight-or-flight response. In a sense, caffeine *is* stress in a cup or a glass.

In the Western diet, coffee and soda are the most common sources of caffeine. You drink a cup of coffee in the morning to wake up. Soon you're drinking two cups, and eventually you're guzzling the stuff throughout the day. It may be a pumpkin spice latte, an espresso macchiato, or some energy drink, but it's still caffeine. Caffeine use is very much like drug addiction, where you need more and more of a substance to get the same buzz. When was the last time you saw a Starbucks that wasn't busy? People have to return to get their fix! And while at the coffee house wiping out their adrenals, these "coffeeholics" are usually also eating foods without the nutrition and vitamins necessary to rejuvenate them. Nor do they engage in beneficial relaxation.

If you want to drink coffee, have decaffeinated coffee or limit your consumption to no more than two (normal size, not a Venti) cups per day. And you should avoid soda altogether, including diet sodas, due to the particularly nasty combination of caffeine, added chemicals, and sugar or artificial sweeteners.

Another way we stress our adrenals is by repeatedly eating foods we're sensitive to. Detection and elimination of food allergies, or more accurately sensitivities (see page 168), is an important way to reduce dietary stress.

Stress reduction techniques—such as yoga, meditation, guided imagery, prayer, and biofeedback—are also powerful tools. Something as simple as making sure that once or twice a day you take 10 to 20 minutes in a room by yourself, close your eyes, and imagine you are in a very peaceful place can be extremely helpful. Take your mind totally off work, e-mail, kids, and problems, and focus, for example, on being barefoot on a beautiful beach with the sun overhead and the waves breaking on the shore. Guided imagery like this, along with deep breathing (see page 61), is a very easy way to prevent stress from accumulating in your body over time.

There is no better stress reducer than a brisk walk two or three times a week for half an hour. Walking is easy and pleasant, it gets you outdoors in nature, and it makes you feel better physically and mentally. It also provides you with some alone time, allowing you to think about what you want rather than just reacting to your environment, as most of us must do throughout the day.

I also recommend reading books that help put things into perspective, such as *Don't Sweat the Small Stuff . . . And It's All Small Stuff* by Richard Carlson, PhD. Sometimes we need a reminder about what is really important and what is just part of the trivial daily grind that we should not get so worked up about.

There are also times when reducing stress can require some difficult decisions. For example, if you're in an abusive or unhappy relationship, have an unrewarding job, or experience a long, nerve-wracking commute to work, you may need to do some soul-searching about whether to make a change. While these kinds of major life changes are difficult emotionally—and usually financially—if these issues aren't addressed and the stress continues, you may never be truly healthy. In the end, what is your health and longevity worth?

5. Make Time for Relaxation and Sleep

The importance of quality and predictable rest and sleep can't be overstated. So many of us are trying to cram too many things into the day. Our Western societies have never fully embraced the need for proper rest. It's always go, go, go! Hispanic cultures have their siestas, and in other traditions, there is often a day of rest, a Sabbath, when commercial activities are restricted. Many so-called blue laws in the United States barring commercial activity on Sunday were religiously inspired but have now largely been eliminated: "Thou shalt create no obstacles to shopping" seems to be the eleventh commandment.

Even our children are falling into a busy work and activity pattern because of pressure from parents and peers to join in an unending number of structured activities, either to keep the kids off the street and out of trouble or to make sure they get into the best college. This and the trend of massive amounts of homework have resulted in very stressed-out and sleep-deprived young people. Is this really healthy? Might the increased incidence of children turning to violence at school or the mall be related to the increasing number of pressured, stressed-out, nutritionally deficient, and overmedicated kids?

Over millions of years, humans have developed the deeply ingrained pattern of being active when the sun comes up and winding down for sleep when the sun goes down. Our circadian biorhythm is set by these light-dark cycles, and we can never be really healthy when we don't respect them. Tissue repair, adrenal and thyroid function, and a multitude of other bodily processes depend on our getting adequate amounts of sleep in a predictable manner at the right time of day. Many modern-day diseases, including fibromyalgia, have been associated with sleep disturbances and the hormonal imbalances that can result. For this reason, working night shifts, especially swing shifts, is particularly stressful to your body and can result in a situation where you may never be as healthy as you might otherwise.

While different individuals require different amounts of sleep, most people need between 8 and 10 hours per day. More importantly, that sleep needs to be predictable and consistent so our bodies can adapt and find a biorhythm. Most of us tend to go to bed too late and get up either too early or too late. I have found that the best pattern is generally to go to bed by about 10:00 p.m. and wake up between 6:30 a.m. and 7:00 a.m. Sleeping significantly less, or more, than this can be detrimental in many cases. It is also worth the reminder to avoid bright lights, including computer and tablet screens, later in the evening to prepare your body for sleep.

People who are always tired sometimes try to "make up for it" by sleeping longer and longer, to no avail. They would be better off getting out of bed and engaging in some moderate activity or movement/exercise first thing in the morning in natural sunlight. Walking around the block a few times first thing in the morning, before showering or eating breakfast, can be beneficial in resetting your body's hormonal patterns, which will increase your well-being in the long run. For information on attaining a healthy circadian hormonal rhythm, once again I recommend you take a look at the book *The Circadian Prescription*.

6. Maintain a Sense of Purpose and Accomplishment

Have you noticed that people who feel they are accomplishing something in life and contributing to the greater good seem happier and more content? This sense of purpose and accomplishment can be achieved through your work, but it can also be generated through service to others of some kind or raising a happy family. I changed my career path from being an engineer to a doctor because I personally felt that I was more suited to help people directly as a health-care provider versus indirectly by designing and working on computer systems. For many of us, a drastic step like that is not necessary. I have also experienced great joy and contentment from something as simple as volunteering to coach youth ice hockey. Helping to teach and mentor kids is about as rewarding as it gets.

I think many people struggle with the issue of whether or not they are making a difference in the world, particularly as they approach middle age. This has certainly fueled the increase in volunteerism and second careers. Often we just become bored with what we're doing and look for new challenges and horizons. While this can be destructive if we constantly up-end our lives, for many people it can be a good thing when done for the right reasons with purpose.

I encourage people to examine their lives—to consider if they are really contributing to the greater good and if they are content with their lives and accomplishments. If not, I always suggest they take steps to change their situations. Sometimes a really major change will be required, such as a career switch or even ending a destructive and unrewarding relationship, but in many cases, it may just mean spending more time with family or dedicating some time to a worthy cause.

7. Clean Up Your Environment

A simple but important step you can take to improve your health and that of your family is to clean up your environment. This includes being aware of the larger environment and what is threatening it and getting involved when you can. But it also includes your immediate environment—your home.

As I previously mentioned, purchasing a water purifier for your home is a wise investment. While reverse-osmosis systems are the best, a carbon-filtration system also works fairly well when maintained properly, and it is less expensive. A water filter installed at the kitchen sink is one commonly used method. But if you can afford it, installing a large-capacity system on the main water feed to your home may be preferable. This way, filtered water will flow to your washing machine, your shower, and your refrigerator's ice maker. By using a water filtration system on your main water feed, your clothes will be cleaner and last longer, your hair will be healthier, and you'll feel a big difference after showering or bathing.

While we can't fully control the quality of the air we breathe, we can help by improving air quality in our homes. A 1999 Environmental Defense Fund study found that more than 220 million Americans breathed air that was a hundred times more toxic than the goals set by Congress in the late 1980s! And for 11 million Americans, the cancer risk from their neighborhood air was more than a thousand times higher than goals set by Congress.[18] The air in our homes, particularly in newly constructed energy-efficient homes that are so tightly built they don't breathe at all, can be full of chemicals from the off-gassing of carpets, draperies, insulation, cleaning fluids, and more. An investment in a quality air filtration system will not only reduce your exposure to potentially toxic chemicals but also reduce the incidence of allergies and asthma. And there will also be less dust, making cleaning easier.

Finally, you can reduce toxic exposure in and around your home by using unscented products whenever possible and refraining from using pesticides and herbicides as much as possible. Newer, organic pesticides, herbicides, and cleaning fluids are available, and I encourage you to use them for the sake of your health and the long-term health of the environment. This is particularly true if you have young children who play in your yard.

8. Keep It Simple!

The old principle "Keep it simple, stupid" is often referred to by its acronym *KISS*. I was taught this philosophy during my training when one of my professors told us, "When you hear hooves, think horses not zebras!" In other words, think about the *common* causes for a particular complaint or symptom before diagnosing a patient with some rare, obscure malady. This is a useful principle in everyday life.

Many of us put added stress on ourselves by avoiding KISS. Do we really need the biggest house we can possibly buy or that 20th pair of shoes? Is burning out your adrenals to acquire more objects that you're told by advertisers you simply must have really a good idea? Do you think they have your best interests at heart? Wouldn't we be healthier if we simplified our lives, uncluttered our homes, and reduced our stress? I think you know the answer to that question.

9. Have Fun

A colleague of mine once defined *fun* as something you do for the experience rather than the outcome. Labeling all the boxes in your storage locker or folding the fitted sheets may be useful and practical, but having dinner with friends, going to see a film, and dancing to your favorite music are all fun. Fun tends to be pointless. That's the point of fun!

I have always liked this distinction and have used it with patients. Many of them realize that they have not been having enough fun in their lives. Even most recreational sports are full of competition, making them less enjoyable. I try and encourage my patients to have some fun every day. The stress relief from regularly engaging in an activity that you enjoy can't be overstated. Even on workdays, you can usually fit in something small, such as listening to a favorite song or playing with a pet. Make it a point to engage in fun activities, particularly with those you love, on a regular basis. You'll be healthier for it! I even go so far as to write out "fun prescriptions" for patients to show their family members so they have an official excuse to go outside and garden, ride their bike, go for a walk alone, or just curl up and read a book.

10. Make Your Health a Priority

My final thoughts are about the importance you choose to give to your health. If you're like most people, your greatest priority is not your health, even though you may say that it is. I can't tell you how many patients I have seen who balk at the very idea of spending money on a bottle of quality vitamins or to see a chiropractor or massage therapist on a fairly regular basis. Yet, they'll think nothing of going out to dinner several times a week or getting their nails done. Many of these same people would spend $800 at the vet's office if their dog had the slightest problem, but would not even dream of spending that amount on a health-related test for themselves.

Why is this? One reason is that we have been convinced—wrongly—over many decades that our health care should be totally covered by our insurance policies and that if something isn't covered, well, it probably isn't all that necessary. This is not true. Bad general health care or disease-based crisis health care may be covered by your insurance and is therefore sometimes perceived as almost free (even though you are paying for it somehow), but quality wellness and preventive health care is not free! At least not in the world we're living in, with a "disease" care system as opposed to a true "health" care system.

People must start looking at their health insurance as nothing more than a safety net against the very high costs associated with serious illness, hospitalization, and surgery. In fact, even things that are covered by insurance are getting less and less free. Look at the increasing deductibles, co-pays, and declining coverage for many services. Patients must come to grips with the fact that if they really want quality care, including preventive and wellness health care, they are going to have to pay something for it. As the old saying goes, "You can pay a little now or you can pay a whole lot more later."

This may mean shifting priorities in order to do away with some of those purely emotional purchases you really don't need and investing some funds into your long-term health. Yes, those vitamins and nutrients may cost some money. The organic veggies and free-range chicken may be more expensive. Office visits to your naturopath, chiropractor, nutritionist, acupuncturist, or massage therapist may not be covered at all. It's all just a matter of priorities. Your health and vitality are your greatest assets. Without them, not much else matters.

Conclusion

It has been a privilege over these many years to be able to help patients struggling through chronic pain and fatigue. I have been incredibly blessed to have met so many wonderful people along this path. It has also been a privilege to try and help you, as a reader of this book, and to hopefully impact your life in some beneficial way. I committed myself to becoming an advocate for a group of people who I felt were being left behind, not taken seriously, and even at times dismissed. Frankly, it really ticked me off and motivated me to learn what I have learned and to do what I do.

I hope you come away from this book equally motivated to get well and to commit yourself to living the life we all want to live—a life full of vitality, happiness, and fulfillment, and free of chronic, relentless pain and fatigue. So please consider what I have suggested in this book. You may have entered this book journey a bit skeptical, and for that I do not blame you. You have likely been through the wringer already in your quest to find out what is wrong with you and recover. But if you have found anything that has helped you along the way to take forward, if you have discovered tools, strategies, and knowledge to be your own best health advocate, then I am very pleased indeed.

I hope that along the way you have really opened your mind to the possibility that you may *not* have this thing called fibromyalgia at all, but perhaps some other real problem, or problems, creating your symptoms. And if, through reading this book, you have determined that you likely do have fibromyalgia in its classic form, you now have options for treating, and eventually recovering from, this disabling condition. Knowledge is power, and after reading this book, you likely have more knowledge about fibromyalgia than the vast majority of doctors out there.

I invite you to use the 21-day Fibro-Fix Foundational Plan every several months if it has helped you; to continue the movement, stretching, and exercise routine; to keep up a daily stress-relieving practice or technique (many have been offered as possibilities); and to review again the 10 steps offered in this chapter to make long-term meaningful and impactful changes in your health.

If there's one most important change to undertake, in my opinion and experience, it's making quality decisions every day about what you eat—and what you don't. Just adopting a whole, fresh, organic food diet—ideally free of processed foods, gluten-containing grains, and dairy—is generally life-changing for those suffering with pain and fatigue disorders of all types. However, by putting together the entire comprehensive plan, as well as being judicious and conservative in your use of medications when they are appropriate (as discussed in the book), you will be on the road to recovery for good. Hopefully you are on that road already.

I would love to continue to help you down that road, so please visit and join our vibrant interactive online communities at FibroFix.com and DrDavidBrady.com to stay engaged and informed. I would also be more than pleased, and indeed honored, to see you in person at my clinical practice if that is possible for you.

Until we meet again.

FIBRO-FIX RECIPES

Section headings indicate whether recipes can be enjoyed by vegans. Use organic ingredients where possible.

VEGAN AND ALL-FRIENDLY RAINBOW SMOOTHIES

Protein powder or Fibro-Fix Detox powder can also be added for variety.

YELLOW SMOOTHIE *Makes 1*

1 cup unsweetened coconut milk

$1/2$ cup pineapple chunks, frozen or fresh

$1/2$ cup papaya or banana chunks

$1/2$ cup mango chunks

1 tablespoon coconut oil

1–2 packets stevia or 1 tablespoon honey or maple syrup (optional)

Anti-inflammatory boost (add one or all)

$1/2$ teaspoon ground turmeric or $1/2$" fresh turmeric, chopped

$1/2$ teaspoon ground ginger or $1/2$" fresh ginger, peeled and chopped

$1/2$ teaspoon ground cinnamon

1 teaspoon ground flaxseed or ground chia seeds

Blend all together.

PURPLE SMOOTHIE *Makes 1*

½ cup cranberry juice or
pomegranate juice

4 leaves purple cabbage

2 stalks celery, roughly chopped

1 ripe pear, cut into chunks

½ cup berries of your choice
(for example, blueberries,
blackberries, or raspberries)

5–6 ice cubes

1" fresh ginger, peeled and
chopped

1–2 packets stevia or
1 tablespoon honey or
maple syrup (optional)

Blend all together.

PINK SUPER SMOOTHIE *Makes 1*

1 cup unsweetened almond milk
or coconut milk

½ apple, cut into chunks

1 banana, cut into chunks

7–8 strawberries

1 heaping handful raw spinach

5–6 ice cubes

1–2 packets stevia or
1 tablespoon honey or
maple syrup (optional)

**Anti-inflammatory boost
(add one or all)**

½ teaspoon ground turmeric or
½" fresh turmeric, chopped

½ teaspoon ground ginger or
½" fresh ginger, peeled and
chopped

½ teaspoon ground cinnamon

1 teaspoon ground flaxseed or
ground chia seeds

Blend all together.

ORANGE SUPER SMOOTHIE *Makes 1*

½ cup orange juice or coconut water

½ cup pineapple chunks

½ cup mango chunks

1 orange

½ sweet potato, cooked and chopped

1–2 packets stevia or 1 tablespoon honey or maple syrup (optional)

Anti-inflammatory boost (add one or all)

½ teaspoon ground turmeric or ½" fresh turmeric, chopped

½ teaspoon ground ginger or ½" fresh ginger, peeled and chopped

½ teaspoon ground cinnamon

1 teaspoon ground flaxseed or ground chia seeds

Blend all together.

GREEN TEA SMOOTHIE *Makes 1*

1 cup green tea

1 cup berries of your choice (such as blueberries, raspberries, or blackberries)

¼ avocado

5–6 ice cubes

1–2 packets stevia or 1 tablespoon honey or maple syrup (optional)

Anti-inflammatory boost (add one or all)

½ teaspoon ground turmeric or ½" fresh turmeric, chopped

½ teaspoon ground ginger or ½" fresh ginger, peeled and chopped

½ teaspoon ground cinnamon

1 teaspoon ground flaxseed or ground chia seeds

Blend all together.

GREEN SMOOTHIE *Makes 1*

1 cup unsweetened coconut milk

1 handful greens of your choice
(such as kale, spinach, or mixed
lettuce)

1/4 avocado

1 kiwifruit

1 ripe pear, cut into chunks

5–6 ice cubes

1–2 packets stevia or
1 tablespoon honey or
maple syrup (optional)

**Anti-inflammatory boost
(add one or all)**

1/2 teaspoon ground turmeric or
1/2" fresh turmeric, chopped

1/2 teaspoon ground ginger or
1/2" fresh ginger, peeled and
chopped

1/2 teaspoon ground cinnamon

1 teaspoon ground flaxseed or
ground chia seeds

Blend all together.

MELON AND GREEN SMOOTHIE *Makes 1*

1 cup unsweetened almond milk

1 banana, cut into chunks

1/3 cup cubed watermelon

1/3 cup cubed cantaloupe

1/3 cup cubed honeydew melon

1 handful greens of your choice
(such as spinach or kale)

5–6 ice cubes

**Anti-inflammatory boost
(add one or all)**

1/2 teaspoon ground turmeric or
1/2" fresh turmeric, chopped

1/2 teaspoon ground ginger or
1/2" fresh ginger, peeled and
chopped

1/2 teaspoon ground cinnamon

1 teaspoon ground flaxseed or
ground chia seeds

Blend all together.

PUMPKIN SMOOTHIE *Makes 1*

1 cup unsweetened almond milk

1 handful greens of your choice (such as spinach or kale)

1/2 cup pumpkin, fresh or canned

4–5 baby carrots

1 banana, cut into chunks

1/2 teaspoon ground cinnamon

1/2 teaspoon ground ginger or 1/2" fresh ginger, peeled and chopped

1 teaspoon ground flaxseed or ground chia seeds

Blend all together.

CHOCOLATE-ALMOND SMOOTHIE *Makes 1*

1 cup unsweetened almond milk

1/2 banana, cut into chunks

1 tablespoon almond butter

1 1/2 tablespoons raw cacao powder

1 teaspoon vanilla extract

1 teaspoon ground chia seeds

5–6 ice cubes

1–2 packets stevia or 1 tablespoon honey or maple syrup (optional)

Blend all together.

NONVEGAN BREAKFAST RECIPES

FRIED EGG WRAPS   *Makes 1–2*

2 medium to large leaves romaine lettuce

2 slices nitrate-free ham or turkey

$1/2$ teaspoon coconut oil

2 eggs

Drizzle of olive oil

Salt and ground black pepper to taste

Sliced tomatoes and avocado on the side

1. Prepare the wraps by laying out the romaine leaves flat. Put one slice of ham or turkey on each piece of lettuce.

2. In a medium skillet over medium-high heat, warm the coconut oil until melted. Cook the eggs to your liking.

3. Slide one egg on top of each ham or turkey slice. Drizzle a little olive oil on top of each egg. Sprinkle with the salt and pepper. Carefully fold the lettuce leaves over the top of the ham or turkey and eggs to make a wrap.

4. Serve with the tomatoes and avocado.

FIESTA MORNING SCRAMBLE *Makes 2 servings*

2 tablespoons coconut oil, divided

1/2 onion, chopped (about 1/4 cup)

1 small bell pepper, chopped (about 1/4 cup)

1/4 cup shredded purple or green cabbage

1 clove garlic, minced

4 eggs

1/2 cup chickpeas, rinsed and drained

1/2 teaspoon ground cumin

1/4 teaspoon ground red pepper

1/4 teaspoon smoked paprika

1/8 teaspoon ground turmeric

Salt and ground black pepper to taste

1 tomato, chopped (about 1/4 cup)

1 avocado, sliced

Chopped fresh cilantro

Lime juice

Fresh salsa on the side

1. In a medium skillet over medium heat, warm 1 tablespoon of the oil. Cook the onion, bell pepper, cabbage, and garlic, stirring regularly, for 5 minutes, or until the onion begins to soften.

2. Meanwhile, in a measuring cup, whisk the eggs.

3. Add the chickpeas, cumin, red pepper, smoked paprika, turmeric, salt, black pepper, and the remaining 1 tablespoon oil to the skillet. Stir to evenly distribute and cook for several minutes, or until the mixture is heated through.

4. Add in the eggs and tomato and cook 2 to 3 minutes, or until the eggs are set.

5. Top with the avocado slices. Sprinkle with a touch more paprika (if desired) and the cilantro. Add a squeeze of lime juice. Serve with the salsa.

Timesaver Tip

Prepackaged veggie blends (for example, Trader Joe's Healthy 8 Chopped Veggie Mix) work great. Just replace the onion, bell pepper, and cabbage with 1/2 of the package of veggie mix.

THE BEST GLUTEN-FREE PANCAKES
(SECRET BRADY FAMILY RECIPE) *Makes 8–10*

Liquid Ingredients

1½ cups unsweetened coconut milk

2 tablespoons grape-seed oil

1 teaspoon vanilla extract

2 tablespoons honey

¼ cup almond butter

2 eggs

Dry Ingredients

½ cup ground chia seeds

¼ cup gluten-free pancake mix

¼ cup plus 2 additional tablespoons coconut flour

For the griddle: 2 tablespoons coconut oil, melted

1. Preheat the griddle to medium-low heat. (Gluten-free can burn easily, so use a lower heat.)

2. In a blender, combine all the liquid ingredients. Blend for 15 seconds. Add the dry ingredients. Blend for 15 seconds, or until blended. Add a bit more of the flour, if needed, or if too thick, add more of the coconut milk. It should be like cake batter, not too thick but thin enough to pour onto the griddle.

3. Add the oil to the griddle. Pour the batter onto the griddle in the desired pancake size and cook for 4 to 5 minutes, or until the edges are slightly firm. Flip and cook for 2 minutes, or until the edges are firm.

4. Enjoy with real maple syrup served on the side.

VEGAN AND ALL-FRIENDLY
BREAKFAST RECIPES

STEEL-CUT OATS AND QUINOA
HOT BREAKFAST CEREAL *Makes 4 servings*

$\frac{1}{2}$ cup gluten-free steel-cut oats

$\frac{1}{2}$ cup quinoa

2 cups unsweetened coconut milk

2 cups water (or 2 more cups coconut milk)

$\frac{1}{4}$ cup maple syrup or 1 tablespoon Simple Maple-Flavored Stevia Syrup (see next page)

Optional Toppings

$\frac{1}{4}$ cup coconut flakes

$\frac{1}{4}$ cup walnuts, pecans, or almonds, chopped

$\frac{1}{2}$ cup berries, chopped apple, chopped banana, or fruit of your choice

Sweet "Stevia Candied" Walnuts (see next page)

1. In a small saucepan over medium heat, combine the oats, quinoa, coconut milk, and water or more coconut milk and bring to a boil. Reduce the heat to medium-low and simmer for 18 to 20 minutes, or until thick and creamy. Stir occasionally to keep from sticking to the saucepan.

2. Stir in the maple syrup or stevia syrup and transfer to 4 bowls.

3. Stir in your choice of toppings (and another drizzle of maple syrup or stevia syrup to taste, if you'd like).

SWEET "STEVIA CANDIED" WALNUTS *Makes 4–6 servings*

1 tablespoon coconut oil

2 cups raw walnuts

2 tablespoons Simple Maple-Flavored Stevia Syrup (see below)

1. In a large skillet over medium-high heat, warm the oil. Cook the walnuts, stirring often, for about 2 minutes, being careful not to burn them.

2. Reduce the heat to medium and add the stevia syrup (make sure the overhead fan is on as the syrup may smoke up temporarily), stirring frequently, for about 2 minutes, or until the nuts absorb the syrup.

3. Pour onto a plate and let cool. Enjoy over salads, in hot breakfast cereal, or just plain for a yummy snack.

SIMPLE MAPLE-FLAVORED STEVIA SYRUP

1 teaspoon natural maple flavoring plus more if desired

1 bottle (16 ounces) stevia simple syrup (NuNaturals makes stevia syrup)

Add the maple flavoring to the bottle of stevia simple syrup. Shake it up. Add a bit more flavor if needed until desired maple flavor. This syrup is much thinner than regular maple syrup, but it is a nice low-calorie alternative to use sparingly on pancakes, waffles, cereals, or wherever you would drizzle maple syrup.

VEGAN FIESTA MORNING SCRAMBLE *Makes 2 servings*

2 tablespoons coconut oil, divided

$\frac{1}{2}$ onion, chopped
(about $\frac{1}{4}$ cup)

1 small bell pepper, chopped
(about $\frac{1}{4}$ cup)

$\frac{1}{4}$ cup shredded purple or green cabbage

1 clove garlic, minced

1 can (14–19 ounces) chickpeas, rinsed and drained

$\frac{1}{2}$ teaspoon ground cumin

$\frac{1}{4}$ teaspoon ground red pepper

$\frac{1}{4}$ teaspoon smoked paprika

$\frac{1}{8}$ teaspoon ground turmeric

Salt and ground black pepper to taste

1 tomato, chopped
(about $\frac{1}{4}$ cup)

1 avocado, sliced

Chopped fresh cilantro

Lime juice

Fresh salsa on the side

1. In a medium skillet over medium heat, warm 1 tablespoon of the oil. Cook the onion, bell pepper, cabbage, and garlic, stirring regularly, for 5 minutes, or until the onion begins to soften.

2. Meanwhile, in a food processor, pour $\frac{1}{2}$ of the chickpeas and pulse until almost mashed (or use a fork if you do not have a food processer). Scrape out the almost mashed chickpeas with a rubber scraper into the skillet. Add the unmashed chickpeas, cumin, red pepper, smoked paprika, turmeric, salt, black pepper, and the remaining 1 tablespoon oil and stir to evenly distribute. Cook for several minutes, or until the mixture is heated through. Add in the tomato and cook for 1 to 2 minutes, or until slightly softened.

3. Top with the avocado slices. Sprinkle with a touch more paprika (if desired) and the cilantro. Add a squeeze of lime juice. Serve with the salsa.

Timesaver Tip
Prepackaged veggie blends (for example, Trader Joe's Healthy 8 Chopped Veggie Mix) work great. Just replace the onion, bell pepper, and cabbage with $\frac{1}{2}$ of the package of veggie mix.

APPLE BREAKFAST BARS (OR ANYTIME BARS!)

Makes approximately 8 bars

Base "Crust"

3/4 cup almond flour

1/3 cup Stevia Baking Blend

2 tablespoons ground flaxseed

1 1/2 teaspoons baking powder

1 teaspoon ground cinnamon

1/8 teaspoon ground nutmeg

1/8 teaspoon salt

2 tablespoons coconut oil

1–2 tablespoons unsweetened almond milk

1/2 teaspoon vanilla extract

Apple Filling

1 1/2 cups apple, unpeeled or peeled (your preference) and chopped

3 tablespoons Stevia Baking Blend or 2 tablespoons maple syrup

1 teaspoon ground cinnamon

1/4 teaspoon ground ginger

1. Preheat the oven to 350°F. Line a 9" x 5" loaf pan with unbleached parchment paper or coconut oil.

2. In a large bowl, mix together all of the base "crust" ingredients.

3. In a medium bowl, mix together the apple, stevia or maple syrup, cinnamon, and ginger.

4. Reserve 1 cup of the base mixture and set aside. Lightly press the remaining base mixture into the bottom of the loaf pan. Pour the apple mixture over the base crust and spread. Add the reserved base mixture on top and spread over the apples, lightly pressing down

5. Bake for 36 to 40 minutes, or until lightly browned and bubbly in the middle.

6. Remove from the oven and let cool completely in the pan. Slice the loaf, and cut each slice into thirds to make the bars. Store in the refrigerator for up to 5 days.

AUTUMN PUMPKIN SOUP *Makes 4–6 servings*

1 tablespoon coconut oil

1 large onion, chopped

2 cloves garlic, minced

1" fresh ginger, peeled and finely chopped

1 teaspoon curry powder

$\frac{1}{2}$ teaspoon ground coriander

1 tablespoon red curry paste

$\frac{1}{2}$ teaspoon sea salt

2 cups vegetable broth (or chicken broth if the soup doesn't need to be vegan)

1 can (15 ounces) pumpkin puree

1 can (13.5 ounces) unsweetened full-fat coconut milk

1–2 packets of stevia to taste (optional)

Chopped fresh cilantro

Ground black pepper

Red-pepper flakes (optional)

1. In a large saucepan over medium-high heat, warm the oil. Cook the onion, garlic, and ginger until softened. Add the curry powder, coriander, red curry paste, and salt. Cook, stirring, for 1 to 2 minutes.

2. Add the broth and pumpkin puree and stir to mix. Cover, reduce the heat to low, and simmer for 15 minutes.

3. Remove from the heat and add the coconut milk. Using an immersion blender or regular blender, puree the soup in batches until smooth. If you prefer a sweet and spicy taste, add 1 packet of the stevia and blend. Taste and add 1 more packet stevia if needed. Garnish with the cilantro and black pepper. If you want more spice, add a shake of the red-pepper flakes.

BUTTERNUT SQUASH, CARROT, AND COCONUT SOUP *Makes 6–8 servings*

2 tablespoons grape-seed oil or coconut oil

1 onion, chopped

1–2 cloves garlic, minced

2" fresh ginger, peeled and finely chopped

$\frac{1}{2}$ teaspoon ground turmeric

$\frac{1}{8}$ teaspoon ground cinnamon

$\frac{1}{8}$ teaspoon ground cardamom

1 bag baby carrots

2 apples, peeled, quartered, and chopped

4 cups chopped butternut squash

3 cups filtered water

1 teaspoon sea salt

Freshly ground black pepper

2 tablespoons honey or maple syrup

1 can unsweetened full-fat coconut milk

1. In a medium saucepan over medium heat, warm the oil. Cook the onion and garlic for 6 to 8 minutes, or until tender. Add the ginger, turmeric, cinnamon, and cardamom and cook for 1 minute, or until fragrant. Add the carrots, apple, squash, and water and bring to a boil. Cover partially and reduce to a simmer.

2. Cook the vegetables for 20 minutes, or until tender. Let cool slightly. Season with the salt and pepper. Add the honey or maple syrup and the coconut milk.

3. In a blender, puree the soup in batches, until smooth. Adjust the seasoning if necessary.

BROCCOLI AND GREENS SOUP *Makes 6–8 servings*

1 tablespoon sesame oil plus more if needed

2 cloves garlic, chopped

1 onion, chopped

6 ribs celery, trimmed and chopped

2" fresh ginger, peeled and chopped

4 cups chopped broccoli

2 cups fresh greens of your choice (such as spinach or baby kale)

3–4 cups water plus more if needed

1 teaspoon sea salt, to taste

1 handful chopped fresh flat-leaf parsley

1 can (13.5 ounces) unsweetened full-fat coconut milk

Ground black pepper to taste

Lime juice (optional)

1. In a large soup pot over medium heat, warm the oil. Cook the garlic, onion, celery, and ginger for 6 to 8 minutes. If needed, add a bit more oil. Add the broccoli and greens and stir until the greens wilt. Add just enough water to cover the vegetables. Stir in the salt and parsley.

2. Increase the heat to medium-high and bring to a high simmer. Cover the pot and reduce the heat to a medium simmer. Cook for 15 minutes, or until the veggies are soft. Stir in the coconut milk.

3. Using an immersion blender or regular blender, puree the soup in batches until smooth.

4. Do a taste test and add more salt and the pepper, if needed. Add a squeeze of lime juice, if desired.

HEARTY VEGGIE AND BEAN CHILI *Makes 6–8 servings*

1 tablespoon coconut oil

1 large onion, chopped

1 clove garlic, finely chopped

2 carrots, chopped

1 can (14.5 ounces) diced tomatoes

1 cup tomato juice

1 cup water

1 green or yellow summer squash, chopped

1 1/2 teaspoons sea salt

1/2 teaspoon ground black pepper

1–2 tablespoons chili powder (depending on your liking)

2 teaspoons ground cumin

2 teaspoons dried oregano

1 can (14–19 ounces) black beans, rinsed and drained

1 can (14–19 ounces) cannellini beans, rinsed and drained

1 can (14–19 ounces) kidney beans, rinsed, and drained

1 cup fresh cilantro, chopped

1. In a large saucepan over medium-high heat, warm the oil. Cook the onion, garlic, and carrots for 5 minutes, or until tender. Stir in the tomatoes, tomato juice, water, summer squash, salt, pepper, chili powder, cumin, and oregano. Bring to a boil.

2. Reduce the heat to a simmer. Add the black beans, cannellini beans, and kidney beans and simmer for 20 minutes.

3. Top with the cilantro.

Variation:

1 1/2 pounds grass-fed beef or chicken can be added to this chili for nonvegans. Just brown the meat first, drain, and add in with the beans.

HEARTY VEGGIE SOUP *Makes 6–8 servings*

2 teaspoons coconut oil

2 large onions, chopped

1–2 cloves garlic, minced

4–5 stalks celery, chopped

1 bag baby carrots, chopped

1/2 head cabbage, chopped

1 teaspoon dried marjoram

2 teaspoons dried thyme

2 teaspoons sea salt

1/2 teaspoon black pepper

2 boxes vegetable broth (or chicken broth if the soup doesn't need to be vegan)

2–3 rosemary sprigs

1 bay leaf

In a large soup pot over low heat, warm the oil. Cook the onions and garlic for 4 to 5 minutes. Add the celery, carrots, cabbage, marjoram, thyme, salt, pepper, broth, rosemary sprigs, and bay leaf. Bring to a near boil, and then simmer for 30 to 40 minutes, or until the carrots are tender. Remove and discard the rosemary sprigs and bay leaf.

Variation:

Chopped cooked chicken can be added to this soup for nonvegans.

LENTIL AND BLACK BEAN SALAD *Makes 4 servings*

Salad

1 cup dry lentils (green or brown)

1 sweet potato, peeled and chopped

2 tablespoons olive oil

1 small red onion, chopped

1 can (14–19 ounces) black beans, rinsed and drained

1 yellow bell pepper, chopped

1–2 tomatoes, chopped

1 bunch fresh cilantro, stems removed and chopped

Avocado chunks or slices (optional)

Dressing

Juice of 1 lime

2 tablespoons olive oil

1–2 cloves garlic, minced

1 teaspoon chili powder

1 teaspoon ground cumin

1 teaspoon dried oregano

$\frac{1}{4}$ teaspoon sea salt

1. Preheat the oven to 425°F. Line a baking sheet with foil. Prepare the lentils according to package directions.

2. While the lentils are cooking, toss the sweet potato in the oil and place in an even layer on the baking sheet. Roast for 15 minutes, or until fork-tender.

3. While the lentils and sweet potato are cooking, in a small bowl, whisk together the dressing ingredients. Add the onion to the dressing to marinate. Set aside.

4. In a large bowl, place the black beans, pepper, and tomatoes. Add the cooked and drained lentils and the roasted sweet potato. Pour on the reserved dressing, including the onion, and stir to combine. Add the cilantro and avocado (if desired) and toss.

5. Chill covered in the fridge for at least an hour. Serve cold or room temperature.

SPINACH AND STRAWBERRY SALAD   *Makes 2 servings*

Salad

1 bag (5 ounces) baby spinach, chopped

1 cup thawed raw peas

1 cucumber, chopped

1 cup sliced strawberries

2 mandarin oranges, segmented

½ avocado, chopped

½ cup Sweet "Stevia Candied" Walnuts (page 243), pecans, or almonds

Dressing

¼ cup apple cider vinegar

¼ cup orange juice

Juice of ½ a lime

2 teaspoons olive oil

2 teaspoons honey

1. Divide the chopped spinach into two salad bowls. Place ½ the peas, cucumber, strawberries, oranges, and avocado into each bowl.

2. In a small bowl, whisk together the dressing ingredients. Pour the desired amount of dressing onto the salads. Sprinkle with the nuts.

Variation:

Grilled salmon, grilled chicken, or hard-cooked eggs can be added to the salad for nonvegans.

LUAU CHICKEN QUINOA SALAD   *Makes 6–8 servings*

(VEGAN-FRIENDLY WITHOUT THE CHICKEN OPTION)

4 cups water

2 cups quinoa

2 tablespoons olive oil

2 tablespoons lemon juice

2 teaspoons ground ginger

1¼ teaspoons ground cumin

1 teaspoon salt

4 cups fresh greens, roughly chopped (such as spinach, baby kale, or arugula)

2 cups cooked chicken breast, chopped (grilled or leftover chicken works great!)

1½ cups macadamia nuts or nuts of your choice

1 cup chopped scallions

1 cup chopped fresh pineapple

1 cup dried cranberries, roughly chopped

1 cup flaked, unsweetened coconut (optional)

1 cup fresh cilantro, finely chopped

1. In a medium saucepan, bring the water to a boil. Add the quinoa, cover and, reduce the heat to simmer for 12 minutes, or until the water is completely absorbed.

2. Transfer the quinoa to a large bowl and allow to cool for 5 minutes. Add the oil, lemon juice, ginger, cumin, and salt and stir. Add the greens, chicken, nuts, scallions, pineapple, cranberries, and coconut (if desired) and mix well. Top with the cilantro. This salad is great at room temperature or chilled.

TURKISH GRILLED CHICKEN   *Makes 6–8 servings*

2–3 pounds boneless, skinless
chicken breasts

Marinade

1 cup plain whole milk yogurt

1 tablespoon paprika

1 tablespoon ground cumin

1/4 teaspoon ground red pepper

Juice of 1 lemon

6 tablespoons olive oil

1. Place the chicken into a marinade bag. In a small bowl, mix together the yogurt, paprika, cumin, pepper, lemon juice, and oil and pour into the bag. Seal and marinate for at least 6 hours in the refrigerator.

2. Grill or broil the chicken until done. Serve with grilled veggies and tomatoes or as a protein on top of a mixed green salad.

BALSAMIC GRILLED STEAK   *Makes 4–6 servings*

4–6 grass-fed steaks of your
choice or 1 flank or skirt steak

Marinade

1/4 cup balsamic vinegar

1/4 cup liquid aminos

2 teaspoons Worcestershire
sauce

1/2 teaspoon ground
black pepper

3/4 teaspoon garlic powder

2 teaspoons crushed dried
rosemary

1 tablespoon olive oil

1. Place the steak into a marinade bag. In a small bowl, mix together the vinegar, liquid aminos, Worcestershire sauce, pepper, garlic powder, rosemary, and oil and pour into the bag. Seal and marinate for at least 3 hours in the refrigerator.

2. Grill or broil the steaks until cooked to your liking. Serve with veggies or as a protein in a mixed green salad.

SHRIMP, MANGO, AND AVOCADO SALAD *Makes 4 servings*

¼ cup chopped red onion

Juice of 2 limes

1–2 teaspoons olive oil

¼ teaspoon salt plus more to taste

Ground black pepper to taste

1 pound cooked jumbo peeled and deveined wild-caught shrimp, chopped

1 cup chopped fresh mango

1 avocado, chopped

2 tablespoons chopped fresh cilantro

1 jalapeño chile pepper, seeds removed and finely chopped (optional), wear plastic gloves when handling

Mixed greens (optional)

1. In a small bowl, combine the onion, lime juice, oil, salt, and black pepper. Let marinate for at least 5 minutes.

2. In medium bowl, combine the shrimp, mango, avocado, cilantro, and jalapeño (if desired). Add the marinated onion mixture and mix gently. Add more salt and pepper to taste.

3. Serve by itself or over mixed greens of your choice for a yummy salad. Best if marinated at least 5 minutes before serving.

VEGAN AND ALL-FRIENDLY SNACKS AND DESSERTS

EASY HEALTHY HUMMUS *Makes 6–8 servings*

Juice of 1 lemon

1 can (14–19 ounces) chickpeas, drained and rinsed

1/2 cup tahini

2 teaspoons dried coriander

1 teaspoon ground cumin

1 teaspoon sea salt

1/2 teaspoon ground black pepper

Water as needed

1/2 cup pine nuts (optional)

In a blender or food processor, add the lemon, chickpeas, tahini, coriander, cumin, salt, and pepper. Pulse to mix, scrape the sides, and add the water to desired thickness. Blend until smooth. Sprinkle with the pine nuts. Keep refrigerated in a glass container. Fantastic with fresh veggies, such as sliced bell peppers, cucumbers, carrots, or any raw veggies of your choice for snacks.

TURMERIC ROASTED CASHEWS *Makes 2–4 servings*

1 tablespoon coconut oil

1 cup raw or dry-roasted cashews

2 teaspoons ground turmeric

1 teaspoon sea salt plus more to taste

Ground black pepper

1. In a medium skillet over medium-high heat, warm the oil. Cook the cashews, stirring frequently, for 2 minutes.

2. Lower the heat to medium and sprinkle the nuts with the turmeric, salt, and pepper. Cook for 1 minute, stirring frequently (be careful not to let the nuts burn). Do a quick taste test and add a little more salt if needed.

3. Transfer the nuts onto a plate lined with paper towels to cool.

NUT BUTTER–CHOCOLATE CHIP COOKIES

Makes 18–24 cookies

2 cans (14–19 ounces each) chickpeas, rinsed and drained

4 teaspoons vanilla extract

$\frac{1}{2}$ cup smooth, unsalted raw almond butter

$\frac{1}{2}$ cup smooth, unsalted raw peanut butter

$\frac{1}{4}$ cup honey

$\frac{1}{4}$ cup Stevia Baking Blend

$\frac{1}{2}$ teaspoon sea salt

2 teaspoons baking powder

1 cup dark chocolate chips or chopped dark chocolate bar (60%–70%) (or non-dairy dark chocolate chips for vegan-friendly version)

Coconut flour as needed

1. Preheat the oven to 350°F. Line 2 baking sheets with unbleached parchment paper.

2. In a food processor, combine the chickpeas, vanilla, nut butters, and honey. Blend, scrape the sides, and blend again. Add the stevia, salt, and baking powder and blend well. The dough will be fairly wet and sticky. Add the chocolate chips and blend. The dough should be just dry enough to press into cookie shapes. (This dough will cook in the shape of the dough ball, so if you just drop a spoonful onto the cookie sheet, it will bake that way and not change shape too much.)

3. Drop 2" spoonfuls of the dough onto the baking sheets, and then slightly press down with the back of a spoon to make the cookie shape. If the dough seems a little too wet to do this, add the coconut flour to the mix, 2 tablespoons at a time, until the dough is the right consistency.

4. Bake for 12 minutes. The cookies will firm up as they cool.

UNBELIEVABLE FOUR-INGREDIENT
CHOCOLATE MOUSSE *Makes 6 servings*

$\frac{1}{2}$ cup vegan dark chocolate chips or chopped dark chocolate bar (60%–70%)

1 tablespoon coconut oil

$\frac{1}{8}$–$\frac{1}{4}$ cup Stevia Baking Blend, depending on the desired sweetness, or 2 tablespoons maple syrup

1 can (13.5 ounces) unsweetened full-fat coconut milk

1. In a double boiler over medium heat, warm the chocolate and oil, stirring frequently, until melted. Pour into a blender. Add the stevia and coconut milk to the melted chocolate mixture and blend.

2. Pour the mousse into 6 small glass dessert cups. Cover each cup and chill in the refrigerator until firm, at least 4 hours to overnight.

ADDITIONAL RESOURCES

Please join the interactive health and wellness online communities at DrDavidBrady.com and FibroFix.com. You will find informative videos, newsletters, blogs, and forums on FM and other topics, and will have access to professional-grade nutritional supplements, nutraceuticals, and other supportive products designed to help those suffering from chronic disorders and health challenges. FibroFix.com includes the Fibro-Fix line of convenient nutritional products referenced in this book. DrDavidBrady .com provides information on a wide array of health and wellness topics and offers access to the comprehensive Formulated Nutraceuticals line of professional-grade nutritional products.

Note: Dr. David Brady does not offer clinical advice for individual cases online, via e-mail, or exclusively through telephone consultations. However, he does maintain a private practice in Fairfield, Connecticut, at Whole-Body Medicine, where he does accept new patients. After being seen as a new patient at Dr. Brady's clinical practice for the initial visit, remote follow-up management is possible. You can find additional information or book an appointment through DrDavidBrady.com. If you are unable to see Dr. Brady in his Connecticut-based practice, you may consider using the practitioner search tool at functionalmedicine.org to find a health-care provider near you who is trained in the functional medicine approach.

Clinical Practice Information for Dr. Brady

Whole-Body Medicine
501 Kings Highway East, Suite 108
Fairfield, CT 06825–4870
(203) 371–8258 (Ext. 2)
info@wholebodymed.com

Professional Associations and Practitioner Search Information

The Institute for Functional Medicine
505 S. 336th Street, Suite 600
Federal Way, WA 98003
(800) 228–0622
functionalmedicine.org

Other organizations that maintain information and/or search tools on health-care providers trained and certified in integrative, nutritional, and lifestyle approaches to health and wellness include:

The American Association of Naturopathic Physicians
818 18th Street, NW, Suite 250
Washington, DC 20006
(866) 538–2267
naturopathic.org

The American Academy of Anti-Aging Medicine
1801 N. Military Trail, Suite 200
Boca Raton, FL 33431
(888) 997–0112
a4m.com

American College for Advancement in Medicine
380 Ice Center Lane, Suite C
Bozeman, MT 59718
(800) 532-3688
acam.org

International College of Integrative Medicine
P.O. Box 271
Bluffton, OH 45817
(419) 358–0273
icimed.com

American Nutrition Association
americannutritionassociation.org

American College of Nutrition
300 S. Duncan Avenue, Suite 225
Clearwater, FL 33755
(727) 446–6086
americancollegeofnutrition.org

Board for Certification of Nutrition Specialists
4707 Willow Springs Road, Suite 207
La Grange, IL 60525
(202) 903–0267
nutritionspecialists.org

American Clinical Board of Nutrition
6855 Browntown Road
Front Royal, VA 22630
(540) 635–8844
acbn.org

Clinical Nutrition Certification Board
15280 Addison Road, Suite 130
Addison, TX 75001
(972) 250–2829
cncb.org

Chiropractic Board of Clinical Nutrition
1840 Forest Hill Boulevard, Suite 105
West Palm Beach, FL 33406
(561) 402–1596
cbcn.us

Contact Information for Laboratory and Testing Services Referenced in The Fibro Fix

Diagnostic Solutions Laboratory
Featured test panel: GI-MAP molecular DNA-based stool analysis
(877) 485–5336
diagnosticsolutionslab.com

Cell Science Systems
Featured test panels: ALCAT food sensitivity test and adrenal stress profile salivary cortisol/DHEA test
(800) 872–5228
cellsciencesystems.com

Genova Diagnostics

Featured test panel: Organix urinary organic acids test (OAT) and adrenal stress index salivary cortisol and DHEA test

(800) 522–4762

gdx.net

Diagnos-Techs

Featured test panel: Adrenal stress index salivary cortisol/DHEA test (OAT) and adrenal stress index salivary cortisol/DHEA test

(800) 878–3787

diagnostechs.com

Cyrex Laboratories

Featured test panels: Cyrex Array multitissue antibody tests

(877) 772–9739

cyrexlabs.com

IGeneX

Featured test panels: Lyme and tick-borne illness advanced testing

(800) 832–3200

igenex.com

Pharmasan Labs

Featured test panels: iSpot Lyme and various immunology tests

(715) 294–1705

pharmasanlabs.com and ispotlyme.com

Contact Information for Dr. Brady's Favorite Quality-Food Providers

Farmers' Market Search

To find a farmers' market near your home, visit:

localharvest.org

Blackwing Meats

(847) 838–4888

blackwing.com

VitalChoice Seafood

(800) 608–4825

vitalchoice.com

ENDNOTES

INTRODUCTION

1 M. A. Fitzcharles and P. Boulos, "Inaccuracy in the Diagnosis of Fibromyalgia Syndrome: Analysis of Referrals," *Rheumatology* 42, no. 2 (February 2003): 263–67.

2 "Chronic Disease Overview," Centers for Disease Control and Prevention, last updated January 20, 2016, cdc.gov/chronicdisease/overview/index.htm.

3 "The Growing Crisis of Chronic Disease in the United States," Partnership to Fight Chronic Disease, accessed February 11, 2016, fightchronicdisease.org/sites/default/files/docs/GrowingCrisisofChronicDiseaseintheUSfactsheet_81009.pdf.

4 L. Lugo et al., "Living to 120 and Beyond: Americans' Views on Aging, Medical Advances and Radical Life Extension," Pew Research Center, August, 6, 2013, pewrsr.ch/1ehcNm1.

5 "About Functional Medicine," Institute for Functional Medicine, accessed January 27, 2016, functionalmedicine.org/What_is_Functional_Medicine/AboutFM.

6 Ibid.

7 M. R. Lyon, *Healing the Hyper Active Brain Through the New Science of Functional Medicine* (Calgary, AB: Focused Publishing, 2000).

8 Ibid.

CHAPTER 1

1 F. Wolfe et al., "The Prevalence and Characteristics of Fibromyalgia in the General Population," *Arthritis & Rheumatism* 38, no. 1 (January 1995): 19–28.

2 S. Mense, D. G. Simons, and I. J. Russell, *Muscle Pain: Understanding Its Nature, Diagnosis and Treatment* (Philadelphia: Lippincott Williams & Wilkins, 2000).

3 T. L. Skaer, " Fibromyalgia: Disease Synopsis, Medication Cost Effectiveness and Economic Burden," *PharmacoEconomics* 32 (2014): 457–66.

T. Knight et al., "Health-Resource Use and Costs Associated with Fibromyalgia in France, Germany, and the United States," *ClinicoEconomics and Outcomes Research* 5 (2013): 171–80.

A. Chandran et al., "The Comparative Economic Burden of Mild, Moderate, and Severe Fibromyalgia: Results From a Retrospective Chart Review and Cross-Sectional Survey of Working-Age US Adults," *Journal of Managed Care & Specialty Pharmacy* 18, no. 6 (2012): 415–26.

4 K. D. Bertakis et al., "Gender Differences in the Utilization of Health Care Services," *Journal of Family Practice* 49, no. 2 (February 2000): 147–52.

5 D. Buskila et al., "Familial Aggregation in the Fibromyalgia Syndrome," *Seminars in Arthritis & Rheumatism* 26 (1996): 605–11.

M. G. Haviland, J. E. Banta, and P. Przekop, "Hospitalization Charges for Fibromyalgia in the United States, 1999–2007," *Clinical and Experimental Rheumatology* 30, supplement 74 (2012): 129–35.

6 M. J. Schneider, D. M. Brady, and S. M. Perle, "Differential Diagnosis of Fibromyalgia Syndrome: Proposal of a Model and Algorithm for Patients Presenting with the Primary Symptoms of Widespread Pain," *Journal of Manipulative and Physiological Therapeutics* 29 (2006): 493–501.

M. J. Schneider, "Clinical Brief: Challenges with the Differential Diagnosis of Fibromyalgia," *Topics in Integrative Health Care* 2, no. 3 (2011).

D. Brady and M. Schneider, "Fibromyalgia Management—Proper Diagnosis Is Half the Cure," in *Insider Secrets for Treating Fibromyalgia*, ed. D. Rawlings (Nutri-Living Corporation, 2012).

7 "Is Fibromyalgia Hard to Diagnose? Make It Easy See the Latest Research," Health Heal, updated October 25, 2015, healthheal.info/why-fibromyalgia-is-so-hard -to-diagnose.

8 R. Terry, R. Perry, and E. Ernst, "An Overview of Systematic Reviews of Complementary and Alternative Medicine for Fibromyalgia," *Clinical Rheumatology* 31 (2012): 55–66.

9 L. A. Arnold, "Biology and Therapy of Fibromyalgia: New Therapies in Fibromyalgia," *Arthritis Research & Therapy* 8 (2006): 212.

M. A. Abeles et al., "Narrative Review: The Pathophysiology of Fibromyalgia," *Annals of Internal Medicine* 146 (2007): 726–34.

D. Dadabhoy and D. J. Clauw, "Fibromyalgia—Different Type of Pain Needing a Different Type of Treatment," *Nature Clinical Practice Rheumatology* 2, no. 7 (2006): 364–72.

D. M. Brady and M. J. Schneider, "Pain and Fatigue: When It's Fibromyalgia and When It's Not," *Townsend Letter* 351 (October 2012).

10 F. Wolfe et al., "The American College of Rheumatology 1990 Criteria for the Classification of Fibromyalgia," *Arthritis & Rheumatism* 33 (1990): 160–72.

F. Wolfe et al., "The American College of Rheumatology Preliminary Diagnostic Criteria for Fibromyalgia and Measurement of Symptom Severity," *Arthritis Care & Research* 62, no. 5 (May 2010): 600–10.

11 M. A. Fitzcharles and P. Boulos, "Inaccuracy in the Diagnosis of Fibromyalgia Syndrome: Analysis of Referrals," *Rheumatology* 42 (2003): 263–67.

12 "Women's Pain: Common, Treatable and Often Overlooked or Mismanaged," ScienceDaily, January 19, 2015, sciencedaily.com/releases/2015/01/150119082754.htm.

13 L. M. Arnold, "Biology and Therapy of Fibromyalgia," *Arthritis Research & Therapy* (2006): 212.

A. M. Abeles et al., "Narrative Review," *Annals of Internal Medicine* (2007): 726–34.

M. B. Yunus," Editorial Review: An Update on Central Sensitivity Syndromes and the Issues of Nosology and Psychobiology," *Current Rheumatology Reviews* 11, no. 2 (2015): 70–85.

L. Pauer et al., "Long-Term Maintenance of Response across Multiple Fibromyalgia Symptom Domains in a Randomized Withdrawal Study of Pregabalin," *Clinical Journal of Pain* 28, no. 7 (September 2012): 609–14.

14 M. J. Schneider, "Tender Points/Fibromyalgia vs. Tender Points/Myofascial Pain Syndrome: A Need for Clarity in Terminology and Differential Diagnosis," *Journal of Manipulative and Physiological Therapeutics* 18 (1995): 398–406.

15 C. Alonso-Blanco, C. Fernandez-de-las-Penas, and M. Morales-Cabezas, "Multiple Active Myofascial Trigger Points Reproduce the Overall Spontaneous Pain Pattern in Women with Fibromyalgia and Are Related to Widespread Mechanical Hypersensitivity," *Clinical Journal of Pain* 27 (2011): 405–13.

CHAPTER 2

1 J. J. Lamb et al., "A Program Consisting of a Phytonutrient-Rich Medical Food and an Elimination Diet Ameliorated Fibromyalgia Symptoms and Promoted Toxic-Element Detoxification in a Pilot Trial," *Alternative Therapies in Health and Medicine* 17, no. 2 (2011): 36–44.

2 E. J. Pantuck, C. B. Pantuck, and A. Kappas, "Effects of Protein and Carbohydrate Content of Diet and Drug Conjugation," *Clinical Pharmacology & Therapeutics* 50 (1991): 254–58.

3 D. J. Liska, "The Detoxification Enzyme Systems," *Alternative Medicine Review* 3, no. 3 (1998): 187–98.

4 G. S. Kelly, "Clinical Applications of N-acetylcysteine," *Alternative Medicine Review* 3, no. 2 (1998): 114–27.

5 J. E. Pizzorno and J. J. Katzinger, "Glutathione: Physiological and Clinical Relevance," *Journal of Restorative Medicine* (March 18, 2013).

6 "Guided Imagery," Cleveland Clinic, January 28, 2016, my.clevelandclinic.org/services/wellness/integrative-medicine/treatments-services/guided-imagery.

CHAPTER 3

1 M. J. Schneider, D. M. Brady, and S. M. Perle, "Differential Diagnosis of Fibromyalgia Syndrome: Proposal of a Model and Algorithm for Patients Presenting with the Primary Symptoms of Widespread Pain," *Journal of Manipulative and Physiological Therapeutics* 29 (2006): 493–501.

M. J. Schneider and D. M. Brady, "Fibromyalgia Syndrome: A New Paradigm for Differential Diagnosis and Treatment," *Journal of Manipulative and Physiological Therapeutics* 24, no. 8 (2001): 529–41.

2 M. A. Fitzcharles and P. Boulos, "Inaccuracy in the Diagnosis of Fibromyalgia Syndrome: Analysis of Referrals," *Rheumatology* 42 (2003): 263–67.

3 G. A. Kelley and K. S. Kelley, "Exercise Improves Global Well-Being in Adults with Fibromyalgia: Confirmation of Previous Meta-Analytic Results Using a Recently Developed and Novel Varying Coefficient Model," *Clinical and Experimental Rheumatology* 29, no. 6, supplement 69 (November–December 2011): S60–62.

4 M. D. Cordero et al., "Mitochondrial Dysfunction in Skin Biopsies and Blood Mononuclear Cells from Two Cases of Fibromyalgia Patients," *Clinical Biochemistry* 43, no. 13–14 (September 2010): 1174–76.

J. L. Dupond et al., "Silent Exercise-Induced Enzymatic Myopathies at Rest in Adults. A Cause of Confusion with Fibromyalgia," *La Presse Médicale* 21, no. 21 (June 6, 1992): 974–78.

5   D. Dadabhoy and D. J. Clauw, "Fibromyalgia—Different Type of Pain Needing a Different Type of Treatment," *Nature Clinical Practice Rheumatology* 2, no. 7 (2006): 364–72.

6   L. Lourenço-Jorge and E. Amaro, "Brain Imaging in Fibromyalgia," *Current Pain and Headache Reports* 16 (2012): 388–98.

CHAPTER 4

1   L. L. Toussaint et al., "Forgiveness Education in Fibromyalgia: A Qualitative Inquiry," *Pain Studies and Treatment* 2, no.1 (2014): 11–16.

2   J. DaVanzo et al., "A Study of the Cost Effects of Daily Multivitamins for Older Adults," presented at Multivitamins and Public Health: Exploring the Evidence, Washington, DC, October 1–2, 2003.

3   A. C. Raghavamenon et al., "Alpha-Tocopherol Is Ineffective in Preventing the Decomposition of Preformed Lipid Peroxides and May Promote the Accumulation of Toxic Aldehydes: A Potential Explanation for the Failure of Antioxidants to Affect Human Atherosclerosis," *Antioxidants & Redox Signaling* 11, no. 6 (June 2009): 1237–48.

Q. Jiang et al., "Gamma-Tocopherol and Its Major Metabolite, in Contrast to Alpha-Tocopherol, Inhibit Cyclooxygenase Activity in Macrophages and Epithelial Cells," *Proceedings of the National Academy of Sciences of the United States of America* 97, no. 21 (October 10, 2000): 11494–99.

4   P. J. Davey et al., "Cost-Effectiveness of Vitamin E Therapy in the Treatment of Patients with Angiographically Proven Coronary Narrowing (CHAOS Trial). Cambridge Heart Antioxidant Study," *American Journal of Cardiology* 82, no. 4 (August 15, 1998): 414–17.

N. G. Stephens et al., "Randomized Controlled Trial of Vitamin E in Patients with Coronary Disease: Cambridge Heart Antioxidant Study (CHAOS)," *Lancet* 347 (1996): 781–86.

5   M. J. Stampfer et al., "A Prospective Study of Vitamin E Consumption and Risk of Coronary Disease in Women," *New England Journal of Medicine* 328 (1993): 1444–49.

6   E. B. Rimm et al., "Vitamin E Supplementation and the Risk of Coronary Heart Disease among Men," *New England Journal of Medicine* 328 (1993): 1450–56.

7   P. Sarzi Puttini and I. Caruso, "Primary Fibromyalgia Syndrome and 5-hydroxy-l-tryptophan: A 90-Day Open Study," *Journal of International Medical Research* 20 (1992): 182–89.

M. Nicolodi and F. Sicuteri, "Fibromyalgia and Migraine, Two Faces of the Same Mechanism. Serotonin as the Common Clue for Pathogenesis and Therapy," *Advances in Experimental Medicine and Biology* 398 (1996): 373–79.

J. J. Alino, J. L. Gutierrez, and M. L. Iglesias, "5-Hydroxytryptophan (5-HTP) and MAOI (Nialamide) in the Treatment of Depression. A Double-Blind Controlled Study," *International Pharmacopsychiatry* 11 (1976): 8–15.

H. M. Van Praag, "Studies in the Mechanism of Action of Serotonin Precursors in Depression," *Psychopharmacology Bulletin* 20 (1984): 599–602.

8   L. A. Arnold, "Biology and Therapy of Fibromyalgia: New Therapies in Fibromyalgia," *Arthritis Research & Therapy* 8 (2006): 212.

W. Hauser et al., "Treatment of Fibromyalgia Syndrome with Gabapentin and Pregabalin—A Meta-Analysis of Randomized Controlled Trials," *Pain* 145 (2009): 69–81.

9 J. Younger et al., "Low-Dose Naltrexone for the Treatment of Fibromyalgia," *Arthritis & Rheumatism* 65, no. 2 (February 2013): 529–38.

10 M. Loggia et al., "Evidence for Brain Glial Activation in Chronic Pain," *Brain* 138, part 3 (March 2015): 604–15.

11 N. Nikkheslat et al., "Insufficient Glucocorticoid Signaling and Elevated Inflammation in Coronary Heart Disease Patients with Comorbid Depression," *Brain, Behavior, and Immunity* 48 (2015): 8–18.

12 B. Dugue et al., "The Driving License Examination as a Stress Model: Effects on Blood Picture, Serum Cortisol and the Production of Interleukins in Man," *Life Sciences* 68 (2001): 1641–47.

13 J. E. Carroll et al., "Negative Affect Responses to a Speech Task Predict Changes in Interleukin (IL)-6," *Brain, Behavior, and Immunity* 25 (2011): 232–38.

L. M. Jaremka et al., "Synergistic Effects among Stress, Depression, and Troubled Relationships: Insights from Psychoneuroimmunology," *Depression and Anxiety* 30 (2013): 288–96.

14 R. E. Sandu et al. "Neuroinflammation and Comorbidities Are Frequently Ignored Factors in CNS Pathology," *Neural Regeneration Research* 10, no. 9 (September 2015): 1349–55.

15 L. Gerdes et al., "HIRREM (High-Resolution, Relational, Resonance-Based, Electroencephalic Mirroring): A Noninvasive, Allostatic Methodology for Relaxation and Auto-Calibration of Neural Oscillations," *Brain and Behavior* 3(2) (March 2013): 193–205.

CHAPTER 5

1 M. A. Fitzcharles and P. Boulos, "Inaccuracy in the Diagnosis of Fibromyalgia Syndrome: Analysis of Referrals," *Rheumatology* 42 (2003): 263–67.

2 M. J. Schneider, "Tender Points/Fibromyalgia vs. Tender Points/Myofascial Pain Syndrome: A Need for Clarity in Terminology and Differential Diagnosis," *Journal of Manipulative and Physiological Therapeutics* 18 (1995): 398–406.

3 Wilk v. American Medical Ass'n, 671 F. Supp. 1465 (Northern District of Illinois, 1987).

CHAPTER 6

1 V. Chedid et al., "Herbal Therapy Is Equivalent to Rifaximin for the Treatment of Small Intestinal Bacterial Overgrowth," *Global Advances in Health and Medicine* 3, no. 3 (May 2014): 16–24.

2 J. A. Bralley and R. S. Lord, eds., *Laboratory Evaluations for Integrative and Functional Medicine*, 2nd ed., chapter 6 (Asheville, NC: Metametrix Institute-Genova Diagnostics, 2008).

3 J. Castro-Marrero et al., "Does Oral Coenzyme Q10 plus NADH Supplementation Improve Fatigue and Biochemical Parameters in Chronic Fatigue Syndrome?" *Antioxidants & Redox Signaling* 22, no. 8 (March 10, 2015): 679–85.

4 M. D. Cordero et al., "Oral Coenzyme Q10 Supplementation Improves Clinical Symptoms and Recovers Pathological Alterations in Blood Mononuclear Cells in a Fibromyalgia Patient," *Nutrition* 28, no. 11–12 (November–December 2012): 1200–3.

5 I. P. Hargreaves et al., "The Effect of HMG-CoA Reductase Inhibitors on Coenzyme Q10: Possible Biochemical/Clinical Implications," *Drug Safety* 28, no. 8 (2005): 659–76.

6 J. D. Harris, "Fatigue in Chronically Ill Patients," *Current Opinion in Supportive and Palliative Care* 2, no. 3 (September 2008): 180–86.

7 J. Haiqun et al., "High Doses of Nicotinamide Prevent Oxidative Mitochondrial Dysfunction in a Cellular Model and Improve Motor Deficit in a Drosophila Model of Parkinson's Disease," *Journal of Neuroscience Research* 86 (2008): 2083–90.

N. A. Khan et al., "Effective Treatment of Mitochondrial Myopathy by Nicotinamide Riboside, a Vitamin B3," *EMBO Molecular Medicine* 6, no. 6 (April 2014): 721–31.

8 G. E. Abraham and J. D. Flechas, "Management of Fibromyalgia: Rationale for the Use of Magnesium and Malic Acid," *Journal of Nutritional Medicine* 3 (1992): 49–59.

9 D. J. Liska, "The Detoxification Enzyme Systems," *Alternative Medicine Review* 3, no. 3 (1998): 187–98.

10 S. Kalghatgi et al., "Bacterial Antibiotics Induce Mitochondrial Dysfunction and Oxidative Damage in Mammalian Cells," *Science Translational Medicine* 5, no. 192 (July 3, 2013): doi: 10.1126/scitranslmed.3006055.

CHAPTER 7

1 G. Neeck, W. Riedel, and K. L. Schmidt, "Neuropathy, Myopathy and Destructive Arthropathy in Primary Hypothyroidism," *Journal of Rheumatology* 17 (1990): 1697–700.

A. Khaleeli, D. G. Griffith, and R. H. Edwards, "The Clinical Presentation of Hypothyroid Myopathy and Its Relationship to Abnormalities in Structure and Function of Skeletal Muscle," *Clinical Endocrinology* 19 (1983): 365–76.

2 A. M. Kis and M. Carnes, "Detecting Iron Deficiency in Anemic Patients with Concomitant Medical Problems," *Journal of General Internal Medicine* 13, no. 7 (July 1998): 455–61.

3 M. Papadakis, S. J. McPhee, and M. W. Rabow, *Current Medical Diagnosis and Treatment*, 54 ed. (Columbus, OH: McGraw-Hill Education Medical, 2014).

4 T. Patavino and D. M. Brady, "Natural Medicine and Nutritional Therapy as an Alternative Treatment in Systemic Lupus Erythematosus," *Alternative Medicine Review* 6, no. 5 (2001): 460–70.

5 D. W. Anderson et al., "Revised Estimate of the Prevalence of Multiple Sclerosis in the United States," *Annals of Neurology* 31 (1992): 333–36.

6 Ibid.

7 C. J. Willer and G. C. Ebers, "Susceptibility to Multiple Sclerosis: Interplay between Genes and Environment," *Current Opinion in Neurology* 13 (2000): 241–47.

W. A. Sibley, C. R. Bamford, and K. Clark, "Clinical Virus Infections and Multiple Sclerosis," *Lancet* i (1985): 1313–15.

C. W. Stratton, W. M. Mitchell, and S. Sriram, "Does *Chlamydia Pneumoniae* Play a Role in the Pathogenesis of Multiple Sclerosis?" *Journal of Medical Microbiology* 49 (2000): 1–3.

P. B. Challoner et al., "Plaque-Associated Expression of Human Herpes Virus 6 in Multiple Sclerosis," *Proceedings of the National Academy of Sciences of the United States of America* 92 (1995): 7440–44.

C. E. Hayes, M. T. Cantorna, and H. F. DeLuca, "Vitamin D and Multiple Sclerosis," *Proceedings of the Society for Experimental Biology and Medicine* 216 (1997): 21–27.

8 A. M. Landtblom, U. Flodin, and B. Soderfeldt, "Organic Solvents and Multiple Sclerosis: A Synthesis of the Current Evidence," *Epidemiology* 7 (1996): 429–33.

D. C. Hewson, "Is There a Role for Gluten-Free Diets in Multiple Sclerosis?" *Human Nutrition: Applied Nutrition* 38A (1984): 417–20.

9 L. S. Lange and M. Shiner, "Small-Bowel Abnormalities in Multiple Sclerosis," *Lancet* ii (1976): 1319–22.

10 O. F. Ehrentheil, "Role of Food Allergy in Multiple Sclerosis," *Neurology* 2, no. 5 (September–October 1952): 412–26.

11 R. L. Siblerud and E. Kienholz, "Evidence that Mercury from Silver Dental Fillings May Be an Etiological Factor in Multiple Sclerosis," *Science of the Total Environment* 142 (1994): 191–205.

12 D. Bates et al., "A Double-Blind Controlled Trial of Long-Chain N-3 Polyunsaturated Fatty Acids in the Treatment of Multiple Sclerosis," *Journal of Neurology, Neurosurgery & Psychiatry* 52 (1989): 18–22.

13 D. M. Brady, "Molecular Mimicry, the Hygiene Hypothesis, Stealth Infections, and Other Examples of Disconnect Between Medical Research and the Practice of Clinical Medicine," *Open Journal of Rheumatology and Autoimmune Diseases* 3, no. 1 (February 2013): 33–39.

H. Tiwana et al. "Antibody Responses to Gut Bacteria in Ankylosing Spondylitis, Rheumatoid Arthritis, Crohn's Disease and Ulcerative Colitis," *Rheumatology International* 17 (1997): 11–16.

14 A. L. Oaklander et al., "Objective Evidence That Small-Fiber Polyneuropathy Underlies Some Illnesses Currently Labeled as Fibromyalgia," *Pain* 154, no. 11 (November 2013): 2310–16.

15 A. Cooke, "Infections and Autoimmunity," *Blood Cells, Molecules, and Diseases* 42 (2009): 105–07.

CHAPTER 8

1 D. M. Brady, *Dr. Brady's Healthy Revolution: What You Really Need to Know to Stay Healthy in a Sick World* (Garden City, NY: Morgan James Publishing, 2007): 99–117.

2 M. de Lorgeril et al., "Mediterranean Diet and the French Paradox: Two Distinct Biogeographic Concepts for One Consolidated Scientific Theory on the Role of Nutrition in Coronary Heart Disease," *Cardiovascular Research* 54, no. 3 (2002): 503–15.

3 F. Bellisle, "Nutrition and Health in France: Dissecting a Paradox," *Journal of the American Dietetic Association* 105, no. 12 (2005): 1870–73.

4 A. G. Costa, J. Bressan, and C.M. Sabarense, "Trans Fatty Acids: Foods and Effects on Health," *Archivos Latinoamericanos de Nutrición* 56, no. 1 (2006): 12–21.

D. Mozaffarian, "Trans Fatty Acids—Effects on Systemic Inflammation and Endothelial Function," *Atherosclerosis Supplements* 7, no. 2 (2006): 29–32.

5 N. J. Mann, "Paleolithic Nutrition: What Can We Learn from the Past?" *Asia Pacific Journal of Clinical Nutrition* 13, supplement (2004): S17.

M. R. Eades and M. D. Eades, *Protein Power* (New York: Bantam Books, 1997).

6 C. H. Wang et al., "Oxidative Stress Response Elicited by Mitochondrial Dysfunction: Implications in the Pathophysiology of Aging," *Experimental Biology and Medicine* 238 (2013): 450–60.

7 J. D. Fernstrom et al., "Diurnal Variations in Plasma Concentrations of Tryptophan, Tryosine, and Other Neutral Amino Acids: Effect of Dietary Protein Intake," *American Journal of Clinical Nutrition* 32, no. 9 (1979): 1912–22.

8 J. M. Donohue and J.C. Lipscomb, "Health Advisory Values for Drinking Water Contaminants and the Methodology for Determining Acute Exposure Values," *Science of the Total Environment* 288, no. 1–2 (2002): 43–49.

9 M. Kawahara, "Effects of Aluminum on the Nervous System and Its Possible Link with Neurodegenerative Diseases," *Journal of Alzheimer's Disease* 8, no. 2 (November 2005): 171–82 and 209–15.

10 J. A. Baur et al., "Resveratrol Improves Health and Survival of Mice on a High-Calorie Diet," *Nature* 444, no. 7117 (2006): 337–42.

11 I. Gigleux et al., "Moderate Alcohol Consumption Is More Cardioprotective in Men with the Metabolic Syndrome," *Journal of Nutrition* 136, no. 12 (2006): 3027–32.

12 L. Djousse and J. M. Gaziano, "Alcohol Consumption and Risk of Heart Failure in the Physicians' Health Study I," *Circulation* 115, no. 1 (January 2, 2007): 34–39.

13 L. Gunzerath, V. Faden, et al. National Institute on Alcohol Abuse and Alcoholism Report on Moderate Drinking. Alcoholism: Clinical and Experimental Research. Vol. 28, No. 6, June 2004; 829–47.

14 P. C. Hallal et al., "Adolescent Physical Activity and Health: A Systematic Review," *Sports Medicine* 36, no. 12 (2006): 1019–30.

J. M. McGavock, T. J. Anderson, and R. Z. Lewanczuk, "Sedentary Lifestyle and Antecedents of Cardiovascular Disease in Young Adults," *American Journal of Hypertension* 19, no. 7 (July 2006): 701–7.

15 P. D. Chilibeck et al., "Higher Mitochondrial Fatty Acid Oxidation following Intermittent versus Continuous Endurance Exercise Training," *Canadian Journal of Physiology and Pharmacology* 76, no. 9 (September 1998): 891–94.

I. Tabata et al., "Effects of Moderate-Intensity Endurance and High-Intensity Intermittent Training on Anaerobic Capacity and VO2max," *Medicine & Science in Sports & Exercise* 28, no. 10 (October 1996): 1327–30.

16 B. Crettaz et al., "Stress-Induced Allodynia—Evidence of Increased Pain Sensitivity in Healthy Humans and Patients with Chronic Pain after Experimentally Induced Psychosocial Stress," *PLOS ONE* 8, no. 8 (August 2013): e69460.

17 P. J. Gianaros et al., "Heightened Functional Neural Activation to Psychological Stress Covaries with Exaggerated Blood Pressure Reactivity," *Hypertension* 49, no. 1 (January 2007): 134–40.

18 EPA History: The Clean Air Act of 1970. https://www.epa.gov/aboutepa/epa-history-clean-air-act-1970.

INDEX

Underscored page references indicate boxed/sidebar text. **Boldface** references indicate figures.

Exercise. *See also* Stretching and mobility
    exercises
  circadian rhythm and, 228
  in Fibro-Fix Foundational Plan,
    28–29
  in FM treatment, 110–11
  in Functional Fix Plan, 187
  in maintenance program, 222–24
  stress on body caused by, 47
Exhaustion, as FM symptom, 6

F

False fibromyalgia. *See specific conditions
    confused with fibromyalgia*
Fasciae, damaged, 20. *See also* Myofascial
    pain syndrome
Fasting, 30
Fatigue, xiii, xv–xvi, xxiv –xxv, 67. *See
    also specific disorders causing
    fatigue*
Fats, in healthy diet, 213–14
Fatty acids, 207
Fiber powder, 35
Fibro-Fix Detox Supplement packets,
    34–35
Fibro-Fix Eating Plan. *See also* Recipes
  detox shakes, 31–32, 34, 38, 39, 40, 41
  finding products needed for, 35–36
  food and drink guidelines, 36–37
  green and red foods, 32
  menu ideas, 41–42, 42–44
  Morning Brew, 33
  overview, 27, 29–31
  simple schedule for, 38–39, 41
  supplements, 32–33
  typical day on, 33–34
  what to expect on, 37
Fibro-Fix Foundational Detox Box, 34–35
Fibro-Fix Foundational Detox Shake, 38,
    39, 40, 41
Fibro-Fix Foundational Plan. *See also*
    Fibro-Fix Eating Plan
  movement and relaxation component
    basic approaches in, 48
    diaphragmatic breathing, 49
    guided imagery for stress
      reduction, 61–63
    overview, 28–29, 46–47
    progressive muscle relaxation,
      59–61
    retraining nervous system, 59–63
    stretching and mobility exercises,
      48–58
  in multifaceted approach to FM, 86
  musculoskeletal issues and, 122–23
  overview, xxv –xxvi, 2, 25, 26–27
  toxin-lowering lifestyle, 27–28, 44–46

Fibro-Fix Maintenance Diet, 218–19. *See
    also* Recipes
Fibromyalgia Survey, 80–83, **80–81**
Fibromyalgia syndrome (FM)
  adrenal support, 105–6
  brain-feedback technology, 113–14
  calming GABA protocol, 103–4
  challenges of, 6–10
  Clinical Reasoning Guide, 79, **79**
  conditions misdiagnosed as, 2–3,
    69–77
  confusion over, 1–2, 64–66
  conventional medicine and, 8–10
  costs of, 3
  defined, 67–68
  depression and, 109–10
  diagnosing, 17–25, 77–79
  Early Trauma Self-Report Form,
    88–89
  emerging therapeutic approach,
    113–14
  example of program success, 111–12
  exercise and relaxation for, 110–11
  irritable bowel syndrome and, 167–68
  long-term maintenance, 208
  medical mismanagement of, 14–17
  medications for, 106, 107–9
  misdiagnosis of, 13–14, 67–69
  mood support protocol, 102–3
  multifaceted approach to treatment,
    84–87
  overview, xiii
  physical therapy, issues with, 147
  research on, xxiv–xxv
  role of stress or trauma in, 87, 89–90
  serotonin, importance of, 90–94
  serotonin-boosting supplements,
    101–3
  stigma of, 10–12
  sufferers, statistics on, 3–4
  supplements, importance of, 94–101
  symptoms of, 4–6, 6–7, 84–85
  tender points, 19–21, **20**
  unanswered questions regarding,
    xv–xvi
  uniqueness of sufferers, xxvi
Fight-or-flight response, 59, 105, 163, 166
Filtered water, 46, 219–20, 229
Fingers, signs of scleroderma in, 204
5-hydroxyindoleacetate (5-HIAA),
    175–76, **176**
5-hydroxytryptophan (5-HTP), 102, 103,
    104
Fluid consumption, proper, 217–20. *See
    also* Water consumption
Fluoridation, tap water, 219
Fluoxetine (Prozac/Sarafem), 108
FM. *See* Fibromyalgia syndrome

Foam rollers
  movement and strengthening routine,
    125 37
  overview, 123–25
Folate, 176
Food sensitivities, 29–30, 168–69, **169**,
    182–83
Forgiveness therapy, 90
Foundational program. *See* Fibro-Fix
    Foundational Plan
Free radicals, 32
Free-range animals, 213
Free thyroid hormones, 162
Fresh foods, in healthy diet, 211–12
Fruit, 42, 212–13
Fun, in maintenance program, 230–31
Functional disorders
  adrenal glands, effects of stress on,
    166
  chemical and food sensitivities,
    182–83
  diagnosing, 70–72
  functional evaluation methods, 171
  Functional Fix Plan, 185–87
  gastrointestinal problems, 166–70, 172
  general discussion, 187–88
  long-term maintenance, 208
  misdiagnosed as FM, 67, 68–69,
    158–59
  mitochondrial dysfunction, 172–73,
    179–80
  nutritional deficiencies, 180–82
  overview, 157–58
  reactions to medication, 183–85
  subtle functional hypothyroidism,
    159–66
  testing guide for, 174–78
Functional Fix Plan, 185–87
Functional hypothyroidism. *See* Subtle
    functional hypothyroidism
Functional medicine
  defined, xxiii
  evaluation methods, 171
  focus on functional disorders, 157
  overview, xxi–xxiii
  research related to, xxiv–xxv
  treatment approach, xxiii–xxiv, 187–88,
    200–201, 203

G

Gamma-aminobutyric acid (GABA),
    16–17, 103–4, 105
Gastrointestinal problems
  as FM symptom, 7
  IBS, 5, 77, 93–94, 166–69
  SIBO, 76, 169–70, 172, 176–77
  supplements for, 185–86

Genetic uniqueness, 210
GI-MAP test, 168
Global pain, 4–5, 5, 18. *See also* Chronic
    global pain syndromes
Glucose level abnormalities, 201–2
Glutathione, 32
Gluten, avoiding, 37
Glycemic index, 42
Grain-fed saturated animal fats, 213
Grass-fed animals, 213
Grazing approach to eating, 217
Green foods, 32
Guided imagery, 48, 61–63, 226
Guilt, related to FM label, 10
Gyms, 222–24

H

Hamstring Stretch, 135
Hands-on physical exams, 13–14, 18–19
Hands-on physical medicine, 118
Hashimoto's disease, 162–63
Headaches, as FM symptom, 7
Health, prioritizing, 231–32. *See also*
    Maintenance program
Health care. *See also* Conventional
    medicine; Functional medicine
  challenges in current system, 2
  changes in, xxi–xxii
  crisis-oriented, xx–xxi
  current state of, xvi–xix
  life expectancy and, xvii–xix
Health clubs, 222–24
Heart, signs of scleroderma in, 204
Heart disease, vitamin E and, 97–98
Herbs, 155. *See also* Supplements
High-intensity training, 223
Hip Extension with a Ball, 56
Hip Rotation, 136
HIRREM (high-resolution, relational,
    resonance-based,
    electroencephalic mirroring),
    113–14
Home, cleaning up environment in,
    229–30
Horizontal Shoulder Stretch, 50
Hydrogen and methane breath test, 170
Hydrotherapy, 33, 34, 46
Hypersensitivity, 6, 77, 89
Hypothyroidism, 21, 193–94, 201.
    See also Subtle functional
    hypothyroidism

I

IBS. *See* Irritable bowel syndrome
Immune system, boosting, 206–7
Infections, stealth, 205–7, 205